THE
SPORTS THERAPY
TAPING GUIDE

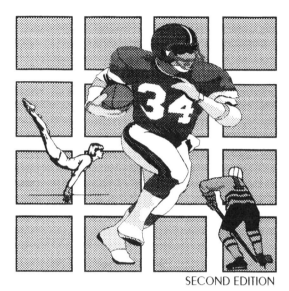

SECOND EDITION

by
Robert Kennedy & David Berry

A
PICTURE
IS WORTH
A THOUSAND
WORDS

Made in Canada

ISBN 0-9695871-0-4

Copyright ©, 1991
Sports- Medics
2373 Urbandale Drive
Ottawa, Ontario
K1G- 3G5
Canada

Authors

Robert Kennedy is the President of FITNESS TECH PRODUCTS INC., a growing company which is involved in the designing, manufacturing and marketing of fitness equipment worldwide. In 1984, he received his honours degree in Physical Education from the University of Ottawa. Over the past eight years, he has been involved in the Sports Medicine field as a Sports Therapist. During this time, he has worked at the University of Ottawa Sports Medicine Clinic with a number of different inter- collegiate teams. In addition, he has been actively involved with several national teams and most recently, in 1990, with the Toronto Argos of the Canadian Football League.

David Berry received his honours degree in Physical Education from the University of Ottawa. He later attended Sheridan College in Oakville, Ontario and obtained a diploma in Sports Injury Management. He is currently Head Certified Athletic Therapist at the University of Ottawa and is an instructor in the School of Human Kinetics. His accomplishments include medical team member with the Canada Winter Games, World Women's Hockey and Ringette Championships and several other national sporting events.

Acknowledgments

The Authors (Robert Kennedy and David Berry) would like to thank the following individuals for their assistance in the development of this manual:

- **Suzanne Real**, for her professional input;

- **Maxime Webb**, for her expertise as copy editor.

In addition, we would also like to thank all our friends and family for their support and encouragement.

TABLE OF CONTENTS

The Sports Therapy Taping Guide

PREFACE

This is a taping manual designed to teach the novice taper
while at the same time offering selected review points for the experienced person.
The manual contains simple terminology in order to reach a broad base of
individuals who are willing to learn or just review the many support techniques
offered.

With this manual we hope to facilitate the learning process via
clear, concise diagrams along with descriptive taping sequences. Through the
experience that we have obtained at University, National, International
and Professional levels of athletic competition, we hope to stimulate some new
thoughts to further the advancement of taping techniques.

THE PURPOSE OF TAPING

Prior to applying tape or elastic wraps, it is important to establish the aim of the treatment. If the goal of using an elastic wrap is to decrease swelling , then the wrap must start below the injury and work upwards to force swelling out. Using elastic tape to secure a sterile dressing would mean that one would have to apply tension that would not compromise circulation. If the aim of a support technique is to prevent a joint from entering a painful range, then one must do simple movement tests prior to the application of the tape. When the tape job is done, one must re-evaluate the movement to determine if the joint is moving in a painfree range.

Too often beginner tapers simply read and follow the diagrams without any thought to what they are trying to accomplish. In addition, beginners forget to make sure that an athlete can function properly in his or her sport with a support technique in place. For example, the use of " buddy taping " does not work in a baseball glove. Always keep the goal of the support technique in the back of your mind when applying tape and elastic wraps.

THE MAIN FUNCTIONS OF TAPING AND WRAPPING

1. To Provide Immediate First- Aid : - Elastic wraps, compression pads and open tape jobs work well in acute injury situations by decreasing swelling and eventually pain. Elastic tapes and wraps are used to provide compression and to hold dressings in place. Tape is also very beneficial for healing structures in that it provides protection but does not completely immobilize a joint. In combination with a proper rehabilitation program given by appropriate medical personnel, tape can facilitate the ultimate return to play for an athlete.

2. Taping To Prevent An Injury : - Preventive taping works well by decreasing the chance or extent of an injury, especially when combined with proper strength and balance programs. Prior to the use of such programs, one must consult the appropriate medical personnel. For certain injuries some strength exercises can actually do more harm than good.

- Preventive taping maintains protection to healing structures on an athlete coming off an injury. Although some injuries can improve with time, ligaments may take many weeks to completely heal. Protective taping can assist with this long healing process while allowing the athlete to participate in his or her sport.

- For athletes who have a history of significant ligamentous injury producing joint laxity, preventive taping can be very useful. This is especially true for athletes competing in high risk sports (football, hockey etc...). In all cases, whichever support technique has been applied, it is important that the athlete be able to function properly within his or her sport.

3. When Not To Apply Tape :   - Although support techniques work well in some situations, they are very inappropriate in others. Taping over any suspected undiagnosed injury in order to allow an athlete to participate, could result in further injury to the athlete. For example, a " running back " with a bad ankle injury may not be able to get out of the way of a hit and as a result could sustain a serious head, spinal or ligamentous injury. If there is ever any question that an injury exists be sure to have it professionally evaluated and rehabilitated. Never let an athlete return to play without written consent from a doctor.

TAPE APPLICATION CONCEPTS

1- The comfort of the person performing the taping procedure is crucial. The taping table height should be such that no bending at the waist is required.

2- When applying tape, follow the contours of the limb involved. Provide good tension on the roll of tape to help eliminate wrinkles.

3- Have the athlete hold the area to be taped in a supportive yet functional position. i.e. " The concept of grasping a ball ", for a thumb tape job.

4- When taping over a muscle or tendon be sure to have the athlete contract the muscle involved.

5- When applying tape, overlap strips by at least one half the width of the tape.

6- Be careful not to cut off circulation with tape strips. Communicate with the athlete during the tape procedure and loosen strips as necessary.

7- To tear the tape, pinch each end with thumb and index finger while applying an outwards force. A quick jerk of the tape will rip the ends more evenly.

8- Have the athlete check the function of the support technique. If supported properly the limb will not enter a pain zone.

SKIN PREPARATION

The skin should be shaved, washed and dried prior to tape application. All minor cuts and blisters should be cleaned, covered with ointment and/ or "Spenco Second Skin " and a band- aid. When taping over nail beds, the use of a small band- aid can be helpful in preventing trauma to the structure. All sensitive areas of friction such as the Achilles tendon, should be covered with a heel & lace pad and skin lubricant. If a heel & lace pad is not available a small gauze pad works well.

The area that is being taped should be sprayed lightly with tuff-skin adhesive spray. This will help the supported technique stay on longer.

Pro- wrap is used to protect skin from the irritation of tape. This is especially true for twice - a - day practices or when there are minor skin abrasions or allergies to the skin. When using pro wrap in conjunction with taping spray, there is no need to shave the skin, however, expect to lose some support.

TAPE REMOVAL

1- Be sure to use bandage scissors or tape cutters so that the skin does not become injured. Dip the end of the scissors or cutters in skin lubricant to facilitate the glide on the skin during the removal process. Follow the body's natural contours when removing the tape.

2- Tape should be removed immediately after its use as bacteria can build up leading to skin irritation.

3- When pulling tape off skin avoid tearing or irritating the skin. Pull the skin from the tape as tearing tape off the skin can cause pain and even injury.

4- If using chemical removing agents to dissolve the tuff- skin spray , be sure to carefully wash the skin with soap and water afterwards.

5- Always watch for signs of skin breakdown such as dryness, redness or infection. These signs could be allergic reactions to the tape and/ or the tuff-skin spray. If allergic reactions occur, stop using the tuff- skin spray immediately. Protect the whole area with pro- wrap to make sure that the tape does not contact the skin. Should a bad allergic reaction occur, refer the athlete to a medical doctor. Athletes who cannot use tape or tuff- skin spray should consider prophylactic bracing.

6- After the tape has been removed , have the athlete apply a skin moisturizer
to the area that was taped. This will help to replace lost moisture and prevent
skin breakdown.

7- For the athlete with known allergies to tuff- skin spray, a hypo allergenic spray such
as " skin prep " should be substituted. If the allergy is to the tape, then perhaps
another brand of tape might be helpful. Adhesive backing will vary in chemical
make- up depending on the tape used.

TAPING REHABILITATION GUIDELINES

When tape is used on a regular basis for prevention of injury, we recommend that the athlete maintain balance and strength for the involved joint.

Using the ankle joint as an example, balance work could be done by standing on one leg and then executing an arabesque gymnastics move (also known as a 747 stand by some therapists). Other techniques for improving balance could be conducted while using a wobble board or a pro fitter. These devices are found in many rehabilitation clinics.

Ankle strength work can be done by doing calf raises and by using rubber tubing to strengthen the muscles on the outside of the ankle. Moving the ankle against the tubing into the position of eversion is helpful. Ask your therapist or doctor for advice before strengthening any previously injured joint.

SPORTS THERAPIST TEAM KIT

BASIC CONTENTS

TUFF- SKIN SPRAY
PRO- WRAP
WHITE ADHESIVE TAPE
ELASTIC TAPE (ELASTOPLAST / CONFORM)
ALCOHOL PREP PADS
TAPE REMOVER
STERI- STRIPS
SMALL COOLER
ROLLER GAUZE
ICE BAGS
SECOND SKIN
HEEL & LACE PADS
MOLESKIN
J- CLOTH
BACITRACIN
SKIN LUBRICANT
HAND LOTION
PROVIODINE (ANTISEPTIC SOLUTION)
BANDAGE SCISSORS
TONGUE DEPRESSORS
MIRROR
NAIL CLIPPERS
TOWELS
SCREWDRIVERS
PEN LIGHT
LATEX GLOVES
COTTON TIPPED APPLICATORS
ASSORTED STERILE GAUZE PADS
KNIFE WITH RETRACTABLE BLADE
EMERGENCY ACTION PLAN & INFO.
PENS & PAPER
ATHLETE MEDICAL INFO CARD
TENSORS (VARIOUS SIZES)
TRIANGULAR BANDAGES
BUTTERFLY BANDAGES

OPTIONAL ITEMS

BLISTEX
DESENEX
EPSOM SALTS
LOZENGES
BULK COTTON
SALINE
SPACE BLANKET
EYE PATCHES
TAMPAX PADS
SUN SCREEN
TWEEZERS
ZINC OXIDE CREAM
CONTACT LENS KIT
SAFETY PINS
FELT

*** QUANTITIES WILL BE DETERMINED BY NUMBER OF ATHLETES ON THE TEAM ***

SPORTS THERAPIST
(PERSONAL ITEMS)

FANNY PACK CONTENTS
(EMERGENCY USE)

LATEX GLOVES (1 PAIR)
4 X 4 STERILE GAUZE (6)
3 X 3 STERILE GAUZE (6)
2 X 2 STERILE GAUZE PADS (6)
TRIANGULAR BANDAGE (2)
C.P.R. MOUTH SHIELD (1)
SPACE BLANKET (1)
PEN LIGHT (1)
6" TENSOR (1)
4" TENSOR (1)
KNUCKLE BANDAGES (10)
ALCOHOL PREP PADS (10)
1/ 2" WHITE ADHESIVE TAPE (2 ROLL)

BELT HOLSTER

UNIVERSAL SCISSORS (1 PAIR)
UNIVERSAL SCREW DRIVER
RETRACTABLE CUTTING BLADE
BANDAGE SCISSORS

Chapter 1

ANKLE TAPE - CLOSED GIBNEY BASKETWEAVE
(RIGHT ANKLE - FRONT VIEW & OUTSIDE VIEW)

PURPOSE: - To prevent inversion ankle sprains.

SUPPLIES: - tuff- skin spray
- 1 1/ 2" white adhesive tape
- pro- wrap
- heel & lace pads
- skin lubricant

IMPORTANT TEACHING POINTS:

SKIN PREPARATION
       AND
BODY POSITIONING

- Spray the front and back of the ankle with tuff- skin.

- Place lubricated heel & lace pads on the front and back of the ankle (See Diagram A).

- Only apply pro- wrap to the skin above the lateral and medial malleolus then figure 8 the wrap to the mid forefoot (See Diagram A).

ANCHORS

- Apply one anchor to the mid arch. Spread the toes apart with your fist before securing the strip.

- Apply three overlapping anchors to the lower leg. These should start low and work upwards but they must not wrap around the muscle belly of the calf (See Diagram A).

SUPPORT TECHNIQUE

- Apply one stirrup on the inside of the ankle then pull it up on the outside. Now apply a " U " strip starting from the inside of the forefoot anchor, travelling below the medial malleolus to end on the outside of the foot on the forefoot anchor (See Diagram C).

- Repeat the above steps, moving the stirrups forward and backward while intertwining the " U " strips. The " U " strips should overlap each other by half the width of the tape (See Diagram D).

13

- Start the figure 8 support strips now
  (See Diagrams E, F, G and H). The figure 8
  must start on the inside of the leg
  (See Diagram E). Rip the tape after completing
  the figure 8 (See Diagram H).

- The heel locks start on the inside of the
  ankle on a 45 degree angle in relation to the
  vertical (90 degree angle) stirrup (See
  Diagram I).

- Follow the Diagrams I, J, K L, M and N   to
  see the proper direction for the heel locks.

CLOSURES

- Finish the tape job by closing up the
  lower leg, starting low and working upwards.
  Overlap each strip by half the width of the
  tape and follow the leg contours (See Diagram O).

- Apply a finishing forefoot closure to seal
  the ends of all the " U " strips. Spread
  the toes apart before securing this piece
  (See Diagram O).

* **N.B.** For an eversion sprain apply four to five stirrups with a neutral force
  (The pull is equal on each side of the ankle). Then apply double
  heel locks with no figure 8 strips. Once this is done, close the tape job. *

OPTIONAL HEEL LOCKS

- This starts on the medial side of the arch at a
  45 degree angle to the stirrup (See Diagram P).
  Follow the Diagrams I, J, K, L, M and N to
  finish this heel lock.

ANKLE TAPE - CLOSED GIBNEY BASKETWEAVE
(RIGHT ANKLE - FRONT VIEW & OUTSIDE VIEW)

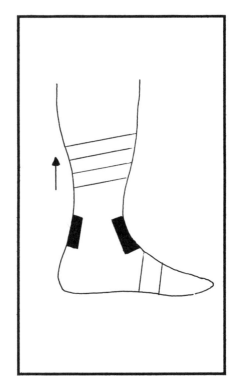

Diagram A

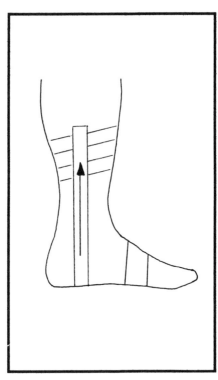

Diagram B

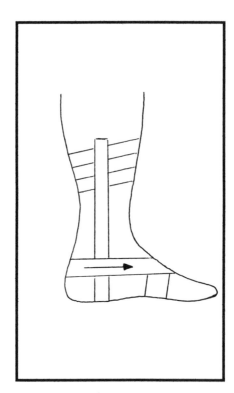

Diagram C

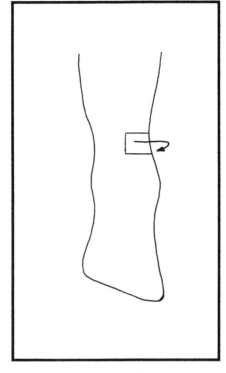

Diagram D

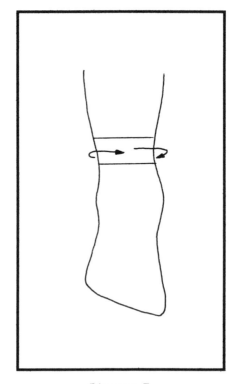

Diagram E

Diagram F

ANKLE TAPE - CLOSED GIBNEY BASKETWEAVE
(RIGHT ANKLE - FRONT VIEW & OUTSIDE VIEW)

(FIGURE 8)

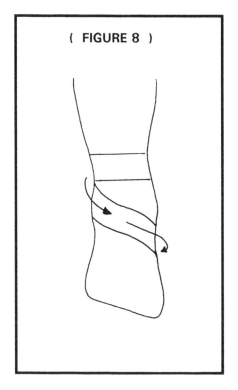

Diagram G

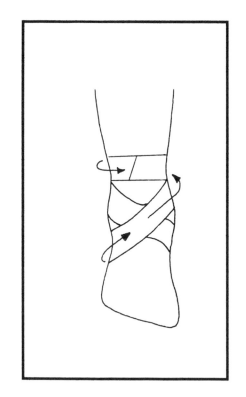

Diagram H

(HEEL LOCKS)

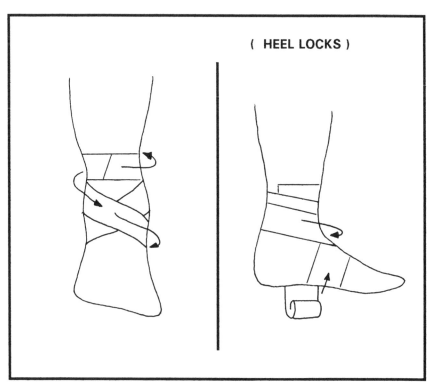

Diagram I

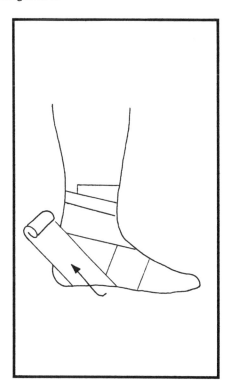

Diagram J

ANKLE TAPE - CLOSED GIBNEY BASKETWEAVE
(RIGHT ANKLE - FRONT VIEW & OUTSIDE VIEW)

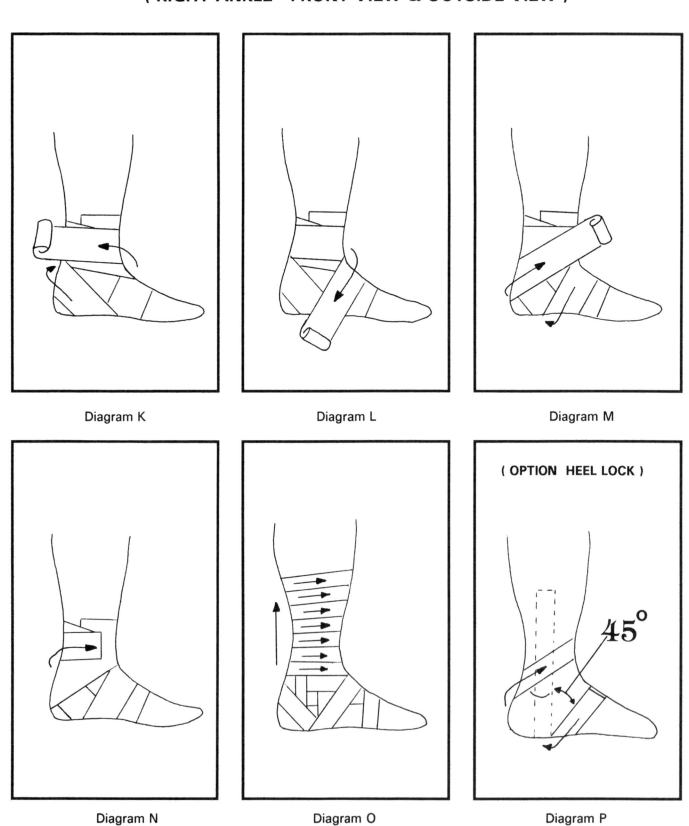

Diagram K

Diagram L

Diagram M

Diagram N

Diagram O

(OPTION HEEL LOCK)

45°

Diagram P

ANKLE TAPE - (CLOSED GIBNEY BASKETWEAVE OPTION)
(RIGHT ANKLE - OUTSIDE VIEW)

PURPOSE: - To increase stability of the lateral ligaments by reducing the chance of an inversion sprain.

SUPPLIES: - tuff-skin spray
  - 3" non- tearing elastic tape
  - 1 1/ 2" white adhesive tape
  - heel & lace pads
  - skin lubricant
  - pro- wrap

IMPORTANT TEACHING POINTS:

SKIN PREPARATION
AND
BODY POSITIONING

- The foot is positioned so that the toes point up to the sky (dorsiflexion).

- Spray the ankle with tuff- skin and place the lubricated heel & lace pads on the front and back of the ankle.

- Secure the heel & lace pads with pro- wrap.

SUPPORT TECHNIQUE

ANCHORS

- Apply one 3" anchor above the belly of the calf muscle (See Diagram A).

- Apply three 1 1/ 2" white adhesive tape anchors to the lower leg just below the belly of the calf muscle (See Diagram A). Overlap these three strips by half the tape width.

- Apply a 1 1/ 2" white adhesive tape anchor to the mid arch area. Spread the toes apart before securing the arch anchor.

STIRRUPS

- Apply a 3" non-tearing elastic tape anchor starting on the medial side of the ankle, level with the white adhesive tape anchors (See Diagram B).

- Bring the strip down then pull up laterally to secure the piece on the upper 3" elastic tape anchor. Repeat two more 1 1/2" white adhesive tape stirrups, one after the other (See Diagram D).

CLOSURES

- Close up the stirrups with two 1 1/2" white adhesive tape strips on the top of the elastic anchor (See Diagram D).

- Complete this option technique with a figure 8 and the heel locks. Close the lower leg but leave the calf belly open (Refer to the closed gibney basketweave tape job).

ANKLE TAPE - (CLOSED GIBNEY BASKETWEAVE OPTION)
(RIGHT ANKLE - OUTSIDE VIEW)

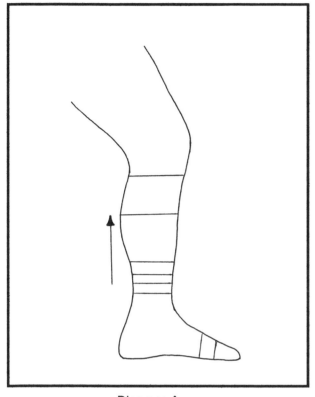

Diagram A

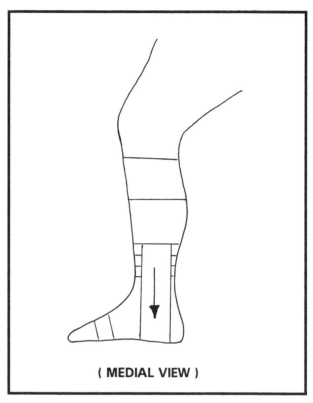

(MEDIAL VIEW)

Diagram B

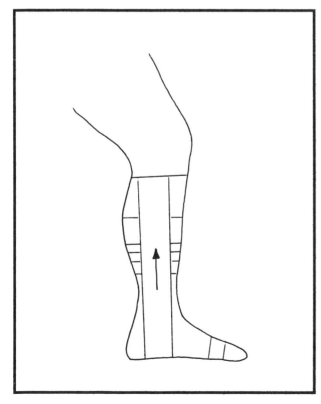

Diagram C

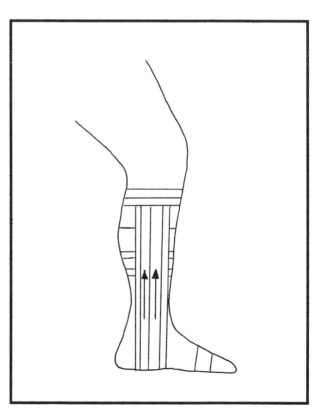

Diagram D

ANKLE WRAP
(RIGHT ANKLE - FRONT VIEW & OUTSIDE VIEW)

PURPOSE: - To prevent inversion sprains with an economical, washable and re- usable cloth ankle wrap.

SUPPLIES: - tuff- skin spray
- baby powder
- 2 " cloth wrap

IMPORTANT TEACHING POINTS:

**SKIN PREPARATION
AND
BODY POSITIONING**

- Position the ankle with the toes pointed towards the sky (dorsiflexion)

- Apply tuff- skin to the front and back of the ankle.

- Have the athlete cover the front and back of the ankle with baby powder to stop friction.

- Place an athletic sock on the ankle.

- To establish the length of the ankle wrap, measure the distance from the floor to an arm above the athlete's head. Cut the wrap to this length.

SUPPORT TECHNIQUE

STARTING POSITION

- Start applying the cloth wrap on the inside of the ankle just above the medial and lateral malleolus (See Diagram A and Diagram B). Go around once to secure the wrap into position.

FIGURE 8

- Begin wrapping a figure 8 by travelling on the inside of the ankle and pulling up on the outside (See Diagram C and Diagram D).

HEEL LOCKS
- The heel lock follows next and starts on the inside of the ankle (See Diagrams E, F, G, H, I and J).

- Secure the ankle wrap with a small piece of white adhesive tape to hold the tension (See Diagram K).

- Use steady tension on the ankle wrap roll to avoid any wrinkles.

CLOSURES
- Repeat the entire procedure once with 1 1/ 2" white adhesive tape. Before securing the tape, fold the edge over to create a tab with which to remove the tape after the sport activity.

- To prevent the wrap ends from fraying, dip the two ends in nail polish or an oil base paint. Do not put the cloth in a clothes dryer after washing. Hang to dry.

ANKLE WRAP
(RIGHT ANKLE - FRONT VIEW & OUTSIDE VIEW)

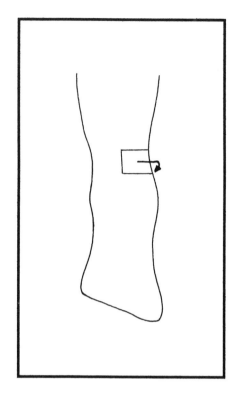

Diagram A

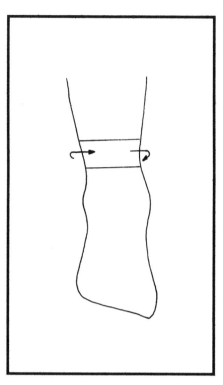

Diagram B

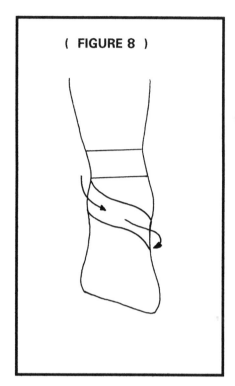

(FIGURE 8)

Diagram C

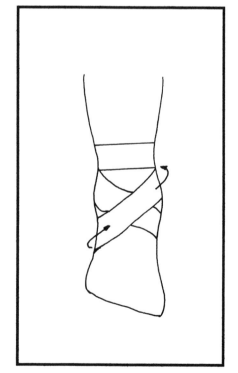

Diagram D

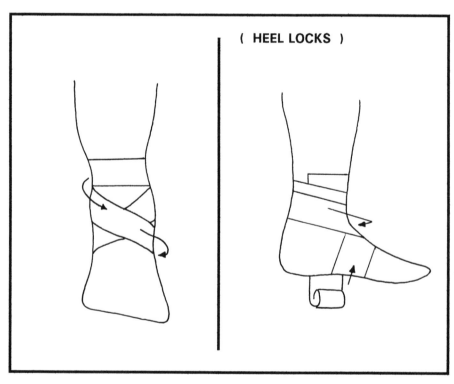

(HEEL LOCKS)

Diagram E

23

ANKLE WRAP
(RIGHT ANKLE - FRONT VIEW & OUTSIDE VIEW)

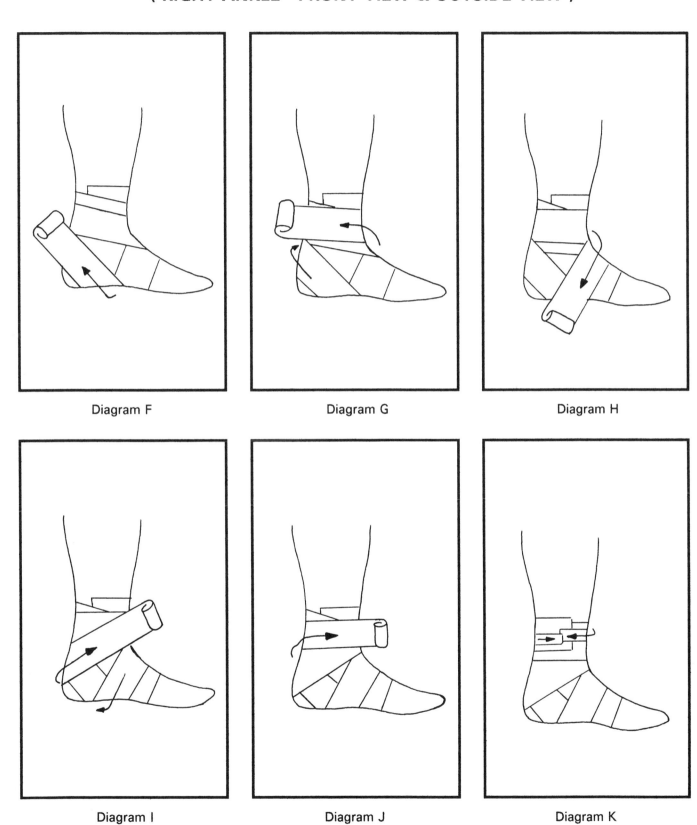

Diagram F

Diagram G

Diagram H

Diagram I

Diagram J

Diagram K

24

ANKLE TAPE - OPEN GIBNEY TAPE JOB
(RIGHT ANKLE - FRONT VIEW & OUTSIDE VIEW)

PURPOSE: - To provide compression and stability to a sprained ankle
in order to assist with the healing process.

SUPPLIES: - tuff skin spray
- pro- wrap
- felt or foam (horseshoes)
- 1 1/ 2" white adhesive tape
- 4" tensor and clips
- skin lubricant
- 2" X 2" gauze pads
- heel & lace pads

IMPORTANT TEACHING POINTS:

**SKIN PREPARATION
AND
BODY POSITIONING**

- Position the ankle in dorsiflexion. The toes should point towards the sky and in a painfree position.

- Spray the ankle with tuff- skin.

- Place a lubricated heel & lace pad on the front and back of the ankle.
- Only apply pro- wrap to the skin above the lateral and medial malleolus, then figue 8 the wrap to the mid- forefoot.

- Place a horseshoe pad on the injured side of the ankle (See Diagram A).

ANCHORS

- Apply one strip mid- forefoot (do not close).

- Apply three anchors to the lower leg, overlapping by half the width of the tape (See Diagram B). Do not apply the anchors to the calf muscle.

SUPPORT STRIPS

- Apply one stirrup by starting on the inside of the ankle then apply one " U " strip (See Diagram D). Repeat this procedure two more times while moving the stirrups forward and then in back of the original stirrup. Overlap each " U " by half the width of the tape.

- Apply two half heel locks to the inside of the ankle and two to the outside of the ankle (See Diagram F).

CLOSURES

- Close the forefoot and heel area with overlapping " U " strips (See Diagram G). Close up the lower leg to cover all stirrups (See Diagram G). By closing at the toes and working up the leg the swelling is forced out of the ankle.

- Seal each edge of the opening down the front of the ankle (See Diagram H).

- Apply a closure strip to the forefoot and to the top of the tape job (See Diagram I).

- Place a 2" X 2" gauze pad between each toe (fold them in half) to prevent swelling to this area. Wrap a 4" tensor around the ankle starting at the toes and finishing at the top of the tape job, by doing figure 8 spirals (See Diagram J).

- Do not have the athlete sleep with the tensor on.

- Icing can be accomplished by placing the tape job (minus tensor) in a plastic bag then immersing the ankle in an ice bath. Protect the toes with a sock before the ice bath.

- Contact your doctor or therapist for appropriate icing instructions.

 * **N.B.** For an eversion sprain apply the same amount of stirrups with a neutral force (the pull on the stirrups is equal on each side of the ankle). *

ANKLE TAPE - OPEN GIBNEY TAPE JOB
(RIGHT ANKLE - FRONT VIEW & OUTSIDE VIEW)

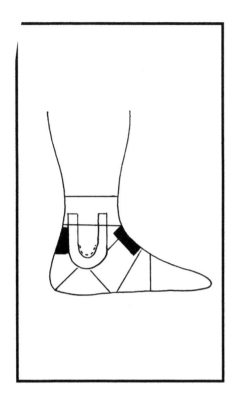

Diagram A

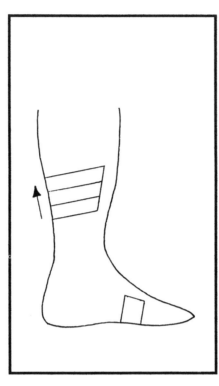

Diagram B

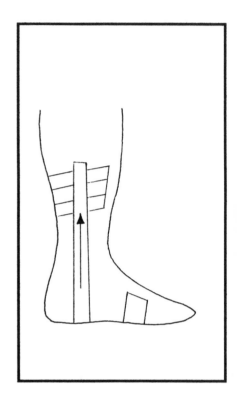

Diagram C

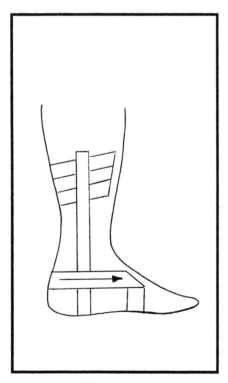

Diagram D

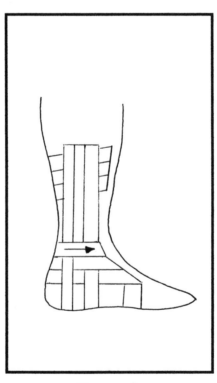

Diagram E

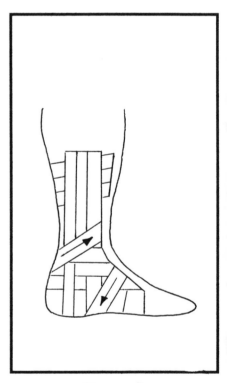

Diagram F

27

ANKLE TAPE - OPEN GIBNEY TAPE JOB
(RIGHT ANKLE - FRONT VIEW & OUTSIDE VIEW)

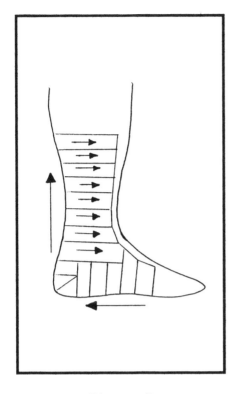

Diagram G

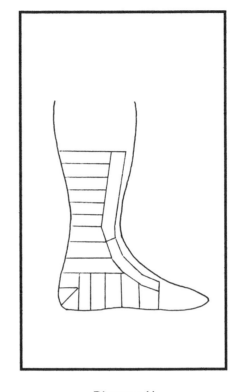

Diagram H

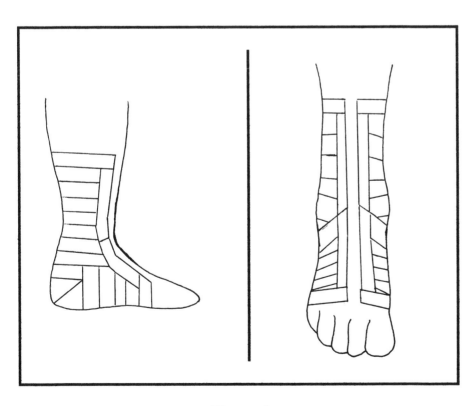

Diagram I

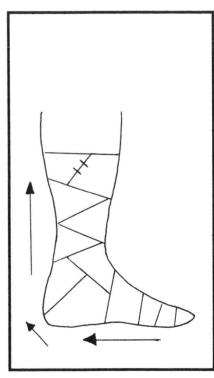

Diagram J

Chapter 2

BUNION (HALLUX VALGUS)

PURPOSE: - To reduce valgus stress on the big toe (MTP- metatarsal phalangeal joint).

SUPPLIES: - 1" and 1 1/ 2" white adhesive tape
  - one small band- aid
  - tuff- skin spray

IMPORTANT TEACHING POINTS:

SKIN PREPARATION

- Shave the big toe and forefoot if necessary.

- Spray the big toe and forefoot with tuff- skin.

- Cover the big toe nail with a band- aid to prevent trauma.

IMPORTANT TEACHING POINTS:

ANCHORS

- Apply a forefoot 1 1/ 2" anchor to the middle of the arch (See Diagram B) and be sure to spread apart the toes before securing this piece.

- Apply two 1" anchors to the big toe and overlap each by half the width of the tape (See Diagram B).

SUPPORT TECHNIQUE

- Pull the big toe into the opposite direction from the bunion position (See Diagram C).

- Apply three 1" white adhesive tape strips starting at the inside (medial side) of the big toe while pulling downwards towards the arch anchor. These strips should overlap each other by half of the tape width (See Diagram C).

CLOSURES

- Apply two 1" closing strips around the
  big toe and overlap these strips by one half
  of the tape width (See Diagram D).

- If the desired tension on the support strips
  is inadequate at this time, detach the strips
  at the forefoot anchor and re- apply
  the tension. Secure the strips in place again.

- Apply one last 1 1/ 2" closure over the mid arch area
  and spread the toes before securing the strip
  (See Diagram D).

- Be sure the support strips do not extend past
  the anchors as it will make closing them
  up difficult.

BUNION (HALLUX VALGUS)

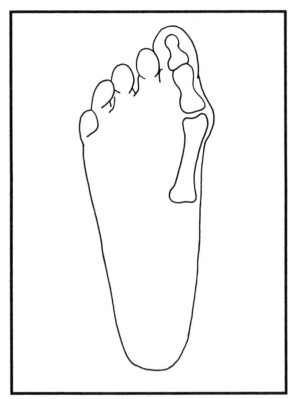

Diagram A

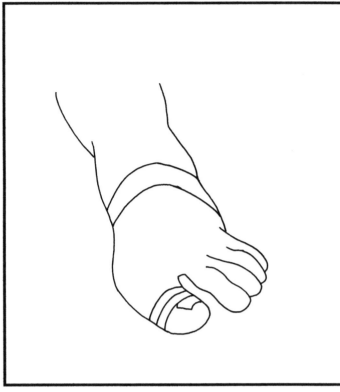

Diagram B

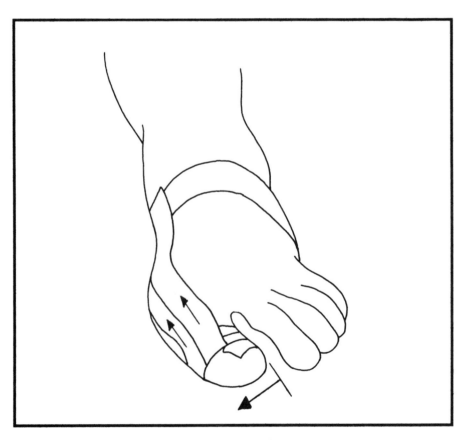

Diagram C

32

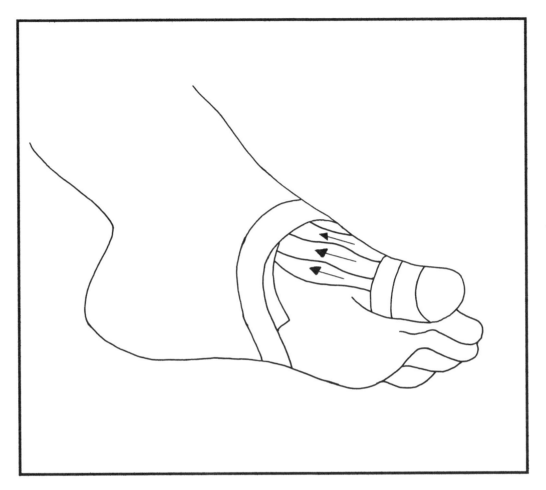

Diagram D

TURF TOE - LEFT FOOT (TOP VIEW)- (FRONT VIEW)

PURPOSE: - To prevent excessive hyper extension of the big toe.

SUPPLIES: - tuff- skin spray
- 1" white adhesive tape
- 1 1/ 2" white adhesive tape
- one band- aid
- 1 1/ 2" elastic tape

IMPORTANT TEACHING POINTS:

SKIN PREPARATION
       AND
BODY POSITIONING

- The big toe should be in a neutral position.

- Shave the excess hair off of the top of the forefoot and big toe.

- Spray the forefoot and the big toe with tuff- skin.

- Cover the big toe with a band- aid to prevent injury to it.

ANCHORS

- Apply two 1" white adhesive tape anchors around the big toe. Overlap the tape by half the width.

- Apply two arch anchors by using 1 1/ 2" white adhesive tape to the mid arch area. Spread the toes apart by pushing upwards with your fingers before securing these anchor strips. This will assimilate the athlete putting weight on the foot.

SUPPORT TECHNIQUE

- Measure the distance from the arch anchors to the toe anchors. On the middle of the big toe, lay on one 1" strip of white adhesive tape with three one inch " X " strips on the top of it to create a checkrein. The ends of the checkrein must be narrow enough to fit on the big toe (See Diagram B).

CLOSURES

- Close the big toe with two 1" white adhesive tape strips (See Diagram C).

- Close the mid arch of the forefoot with two 1 1/ 2" white adhesive strips. Spread the two toes apart prior to securing the closures (See Diagram C).

OPTION

- Secure a strip of 1 1/ 2" elastic tape starting from the arch anchor, spiraling around the big toe (See Diagram D) to finish back on the arch anchor. Close the end with a 1 1/ 2" white adhesive tape anchor. This elastic tape strip is added to the regular turf toe.

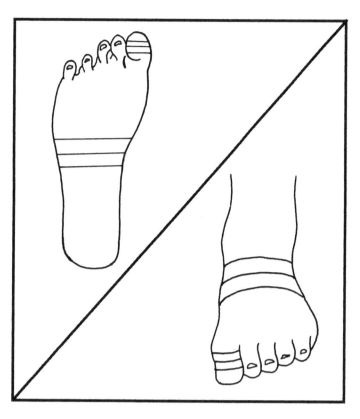

Diagram A

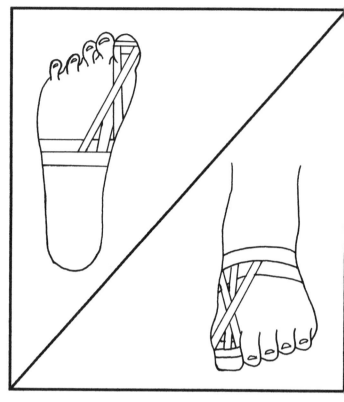

Diagram B

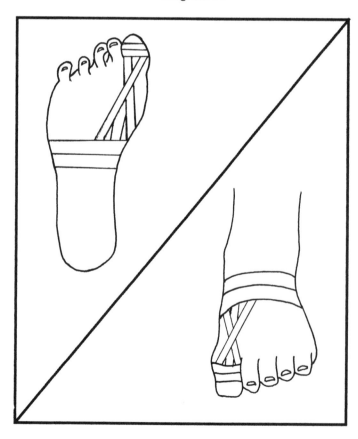

Diagram C

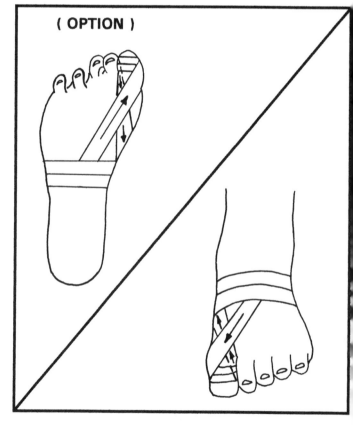

(OPTION)

Diagram D

ARCH TAPING - PLANTAR FASCITIS

PURPOSE: - To be used to support the plantar fascia (arch), and can also provide relief from " Shin Splints " .

SUPPLIES: - tuff- skin spray
- 1 1/ 2" white adhesive tape
- 1" white adhesive tape
- heel & lace pads
- skin lubricant
- 2" white adhesive tape

IMPORTANT TEACHING POINTS:

SKIN PREPARATION
- Spray the top and bottom of the foot with tuff- skin.

- Place half of a lubricated heel & lace pad at the back of the heel and secure it in place with one 2" white adhesive tape strip.

ANCHORS
- Apply one forefoot anchor at the base of the toes using 1 1/ 2" white adhesive tape (See Diagram A). Before securing this strip spread the athlete's toes apart with your fist.

- Apply one 1 1/ 2" peripheral anchor strip by starting on the outside forefoot anchor, continuing around the heel and finishing on the inside of the forefoot anchor (See Diagram B).

SUPPORT STRIPS
- These strips require 1" white adhesive tape.

- Start the first arch strip on the forefoot anchor beneath the 4th toe. Carry this strip down and over the heel pad to finish at the base of the big toe (See Diagram C).

- Repeat the arch strip two more times by having the strip start on the forefoot anchor beneath the 2nd and 3rd toe respectively. These strips should finish near the base of the big toe (See Diagram D and Diagram E).

CLOSURES

- Begin closing the arch support strips by using 1 1/2" white adhesive tape (See Diagram F).

- Begin the 1st closure strip just in front of the heel by starting and finishing the strip on the top of the foot.

- These strips must start on the outside of the top of the foot and then pull up on the inside arch (See Diagram F).

- Continue applying these closure strips while working down towards the toes. Be sure to spread apart the toes before securing the tape strips.

- All the toes should be free to move so do not cover them up.

ARCH TAPING - PLANTAR FASCITIS

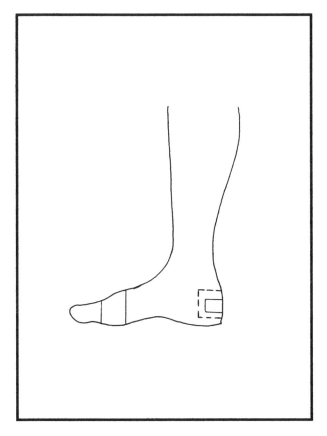

Diagram A

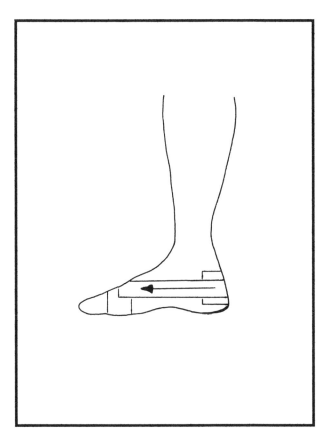

Diagram B

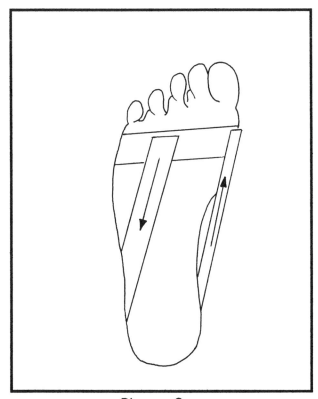

Diagram C

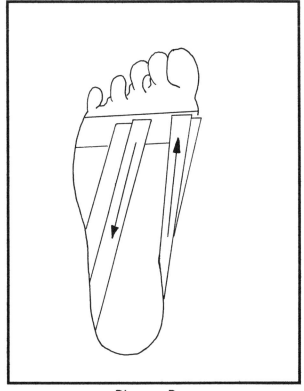

Diagram D

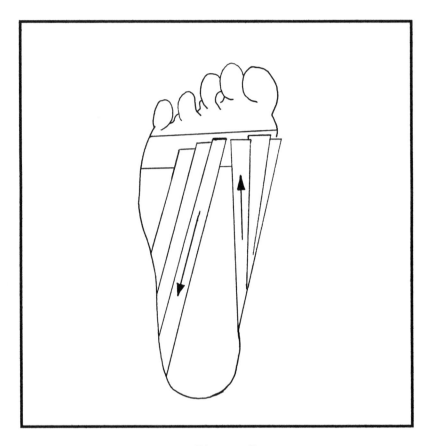

Diagram E

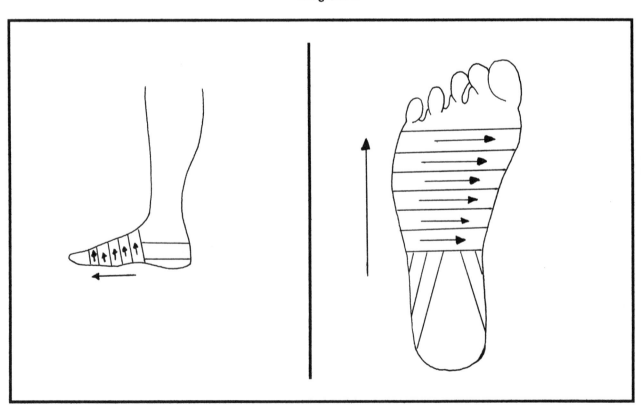

Diagram F

MOLESKIN ARCH TAPING

PURPOSE: - To provide support to the arch and to the foot.

SUPPLIES: - 3" wide moleskin
- tuff- skin spray
- 1 1/ 2" white adhesive tape
- 1" white adhesive tape

IMPORTANT TEACHING POINTS:

SKIN PREPARATION AND BODY POSITIONING
- Spray the bottom of the foot with tuff- skin.

- Have the athlete sit on a taping table with the arch facing the person doing the taping.

ANCHORS
- Secure an anchor around the forefoot near the base of the toes. Be sure to spread apart the toes by pushing on the bottom of the foot. This will ensure that the anchor does not interfere with the normal movements while the athlete is weight bearing (See Diagram A).

SUPPORT TECHNIQUE
- Once the moleskin has been measured and cut (See Diagram B), secure it at the back of the heel then again at the forefoot anchor.

CLOSURES
- Secure the moleskin by beginning one 1" strip on the outside of the fifth toe. Continue this strip down around the heel to finish beside the base of the big toe on the forefoot anchor. Repeat this strip again and overlap the piece by one half the tape width (See Diagram D).

- Place the final closure around the base of the toes to cover up the original forefoot anchor. Be sure to spread the toes apart before securing the tape (See Diagram D).

MOLESKIN ARCH TAPING

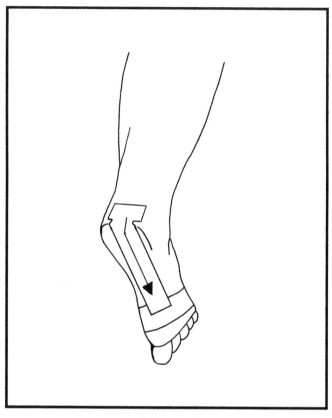

Diagram A

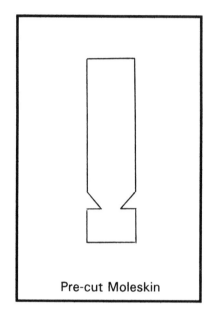

Pre-cut Moleskin

Diagram B

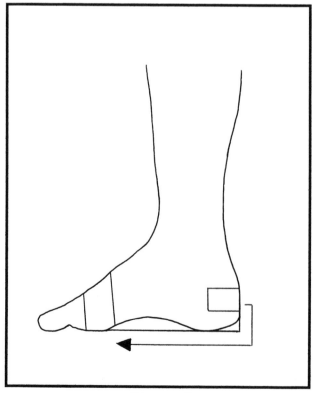

Diagram C

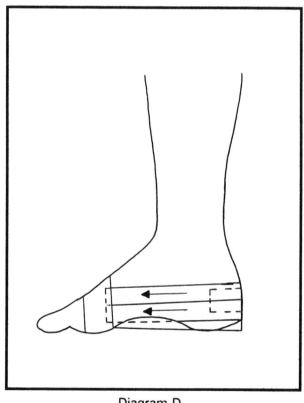

Diagram D

42

ACHILLES TENDON TAPING

PURPOSE: - To provide support for the achilles tendon by limiting extreme dorsiflexion of the ankle.

SUPPLIES: - tuff- skin spray
- 1 1/ 2" white adhesive tape
- 3" non tearing elastic tape
- medium density foam
- skin lubricant
- 3" thin elastic tape (conform)

IMPORTANT TEACHING POINTS:

**SKIN PREPARATION
AND
BODY POSITIONING**

- Shave the lower leg.

- Apply tuff- skin spray to the lower leg.

- Position the athlete lying on their stomach on a table or kneeling on a chair with the ankle slightly pointed (plantar flexion).

ANCHORS

- Apply two forefoot anchors to the mid arch and overlap them by half the width of the tape. Spread apart the toes before securing each strip (See Diagram A).

- Apply three 1 1/ 2" white adhesive tape strips to the lower leg just below the belly of the calf. Overlap these strips by half the width of the tape (for athletes with long lower legs and high calf muscles, do not go more than approximately twelve inches above the heel with this support technique - See Diagram B).

SUPPORT TECHNIQUE

- Lay on a 3" non tearing elastic tape strip on the bottom of the forefoot anchor. Secure this with a 1 1/ 2" white adhesive tape strip (See Diagram C). Pull up this piece while applying tension and secure it to the calf anchors with a 1 1/ 2" white adhesive tape strip.

- Lay a second strip of elastic tape on the plantar aspect of the forefoot. Secure this with a 1 1/2" white adhesive tape strip.

- Measure this piece so that is long enough to be split and secured to the calf anchor (See Diagram C).

CLOSURES

- Close in the forefoot with two forefoot 1 1/2" white adhesive tape strips. Overlap these by half the width of the tape (See Diagram D).

- Close up the lower leg with five or six 1 1/2" white adhesive tape strips. Do not apply the closures to the calf muscle belly as it could cramp or fatigue. Overlap the closures by half the width of the tape (See Diagram D).

* N.B. Fold the elastic tape over on each side of the base of the achilles tendon area and then apply skin lubricant to the achilles tendon to stop any friction.

A heel lift may be used (medium density foam) to give support to the achilles. It is a good idea for the athlete to wear one heel lift in each shoe to prevent any other body problems.

OPTIONAL CLOSURE

- Spiral a very thin elastic tape around the entire procedure from the forefoot upwards to secure the finished technique (See Diagram E for closure).

ACHILLES TENDON TAPING

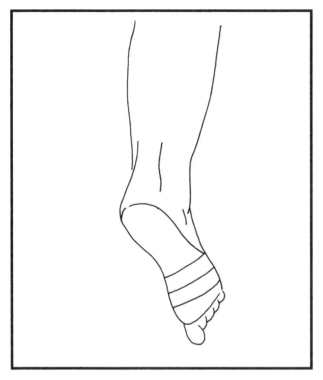

Diagram A

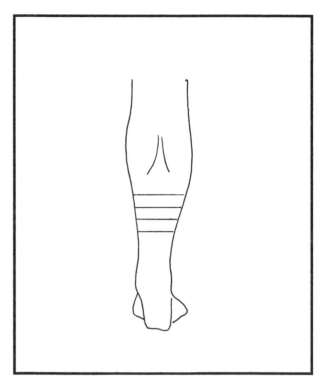

Diagram B

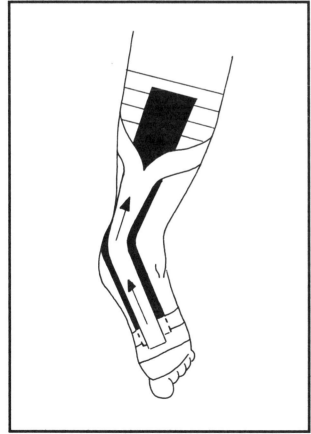

Diagram C

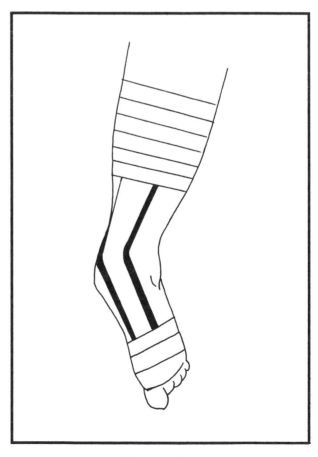

Diagram D

45

ACHILLES TENDON TAPING

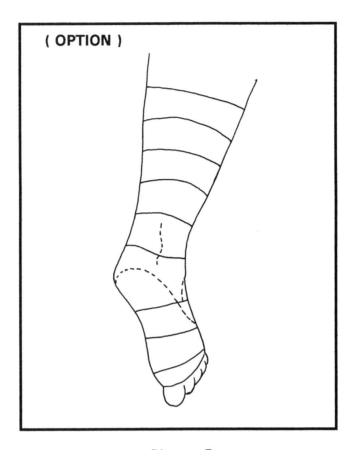

(OPTION)

Diagram E

SHIN SPLINTS - ANTERIOR COMPARTMENT
(RIGHT SHIN - FRONT VIEW)

PURPOSE: - To provide support to the outside muscles of the lower leg due to pain from overuse of the limb.

SUPPLIES: - tuff- skin spray
- 1 1/2" white adhesive tape
- 3/ 8 " thick foam pad

IMPORTANT TEACHING POINTS:

**SKIN PREPARATION
AND
BODY POSITIONING**

- Shave the lower leg.

- Spray the skin with tuff- skin.

- Have the athlete stand on a table.

- Place a small pad, 1" wide and 6" long over the area of tenderness. The use of 1/ 4" to 3/ 8" thick foam is ideal (See Diagram A).

ANCHORS

- Place one 1 1/ 2" white adhesive tape anchor on the outside of the lower leg. This piece starts at the tip of the lateral malleolus and rises up the lower leg to below the muscle belly of the calf (See Diagram A).

- Place another 1 1/ 2" white adhesive tape anchor on the inside of the lower leg. The boundaries for this strip lie between the tip of the medial malleolus and below the calf muscle belly (See Diagram A).

SUPPORT TECHNIQUE

- Begin the spiral support strips on the inside of the lower leg, just above the medial malleolus (See Diagram B). These strips start on the inside anchor, travel behind the achilles tendon, spiral up and over the area of tenderness, and finish on the inside anchor (See Diagram B).

- Overlap the spiral support strips by half the width of the tape.

- Repeat the spiral technique about three to four times. The number of strips will depend on the length of the lower leg.

CLOSURES
- Start the 1 1/2" white adhesive tape closure strips just above the lateral and medial malleolus. All closure strips start on the inside, travel down on an angle to pass around the achilles, and then rise back up on an angle. Tear off the strips of tape at this point. Repeat this " angle down " and " angle up " procedure until the support technique is closed in. This will create a herring bone pattern (See Diagram C).

- Do not tape over the muscle belly of the calf as the muscle could cramp or fatigue.

OPTION
- For extra support use the arch taping procedure in combination with the shin splint tape job.

SHIN SPLINTS - ANTERIOR COMPARTMENT
(RIGHT SHIN - FRONT VIEW)

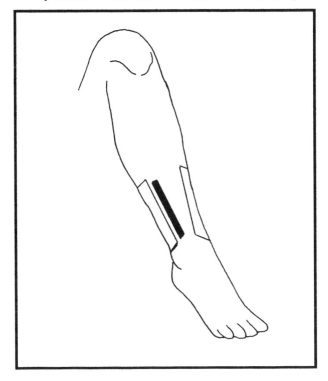

Diagram A

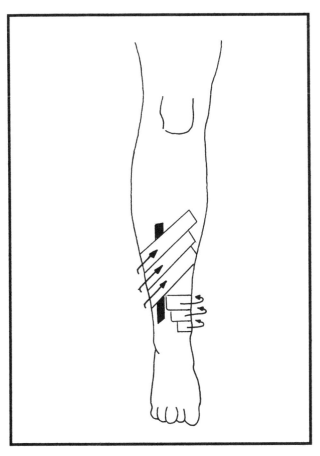

Diagram B

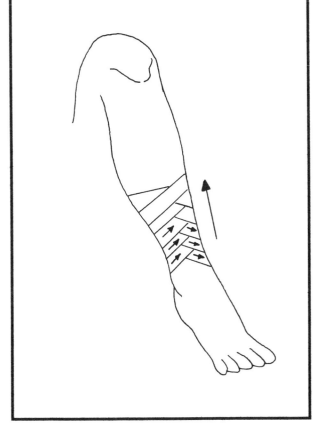

Diagram C

MEDIAL COMPARTMENT SHIN SPLINTS

SPECIAL INSTRUCTIONS

PURPOSE

- To provide support to the inside muscles of the lower leg due to pain from overuse of the limb.

SKIN PREPARATION

- Same taping materials as anterior compartment.

- Move the compression pad to the inside of the lower leg.

SUPPORT SPIRAL STRIPS

- These strips start on the outside of the lower leg then spiral upwards moving medially.

CLOSURES

- These begin on the outside of the lower leg. They traverse downward on the outside of the lower leg and finish by pulling up and over the inside of the lower leg.

Chapter 3

KNEE- MEDIAL COLLATERAL LIGAMENT TAPING

PURPOSE: - To provide support for a medial collateral ligament.

SUPPLIES: - 3" elastic tape
- heel & lace pads
- pro-wrap
- skin lubricant
- 1 1/ 2" white adhesive tape
- tuff- skin spray

IMPORTANT TEACHING POINTS:

**SKIN PREPARATION
&
BODY POSITIONING**

- Shave the thigh and lower leg.

- Spray the entire knee with tuff- skin.

- Apply a lubricated heel & lace pad to the back of the knee to prevent irritation.

- Secure the heel & lace pad with pro- wrap starting just above the calf and finishing mid thigh. The pro- wrap will be secured by the elastic anchors.

- Position the athlete by placing a 1 1/ 2" roll of white adhesive tape under the heel (See Diagram A).

- Once the leg is bent, turn the lower leg inwards.

ANCHORS

- Apply the upper anchors mid to upper thigh using two 3" elastic tape strips. These should be overlapped by half the width and must be applied to the skin (See Diagram B).

- Apply two 3" elastic tape anchors strips to just below the mid calf and overlap each strip by half the width of the tape. These strips must be applied to the skin (See Diagram B).

52

SUPPORT TECHNIQUE

- Start the first support strip on the outside
  of the lower anchor (See Diagram C).

- This strip should traverse upwards crossing
  the joint line but remaining below the knee
  cap. The tape must be stretched to the maximum
  and then applied to the upper anchors.

- The second support strip starts on the inner
  part of the calf anchors. It crosses the
  joint line, rises above the knee cap and is secured
  on the upper anchor. The elastic tape must be stretched
  to the maximum then applied to the upper anchor
  (See Diagram D).

- The third strip travels on the inside of the knee
  going from the calf anchor to the upper thigh anchors
  (See Diagram E).

- Repeat steps 1, 2, 3.

**DEROTATION
STRIPS**

- Start the derotation strip at the calf anchor on the
  front of the lower leg. Pull the strip inwards
  and spiral upwards behind the knee, then
  upwards around the outside of the thigh to finish
  on the upper inner thigh anchor (See Diagram F).

CLOSURES

- Close the lower leg using 3" elastic tape strips.
  Start at the calf anchor and then work upwards
  to below the knee cap. Do not spiral continuously.
  Cut the tape after each turn around the leg and
  overlap the pieces by half the width. Continue the
  closure above the knee and then finish on
  the upper thigh. Close the elastic tape on the upper
  thigh with three 1 1/ 2" white adhesive tape
  strips (See Diagram G).

KNEE- MEDIAL COLLATERAL LIGAMENT TAPING

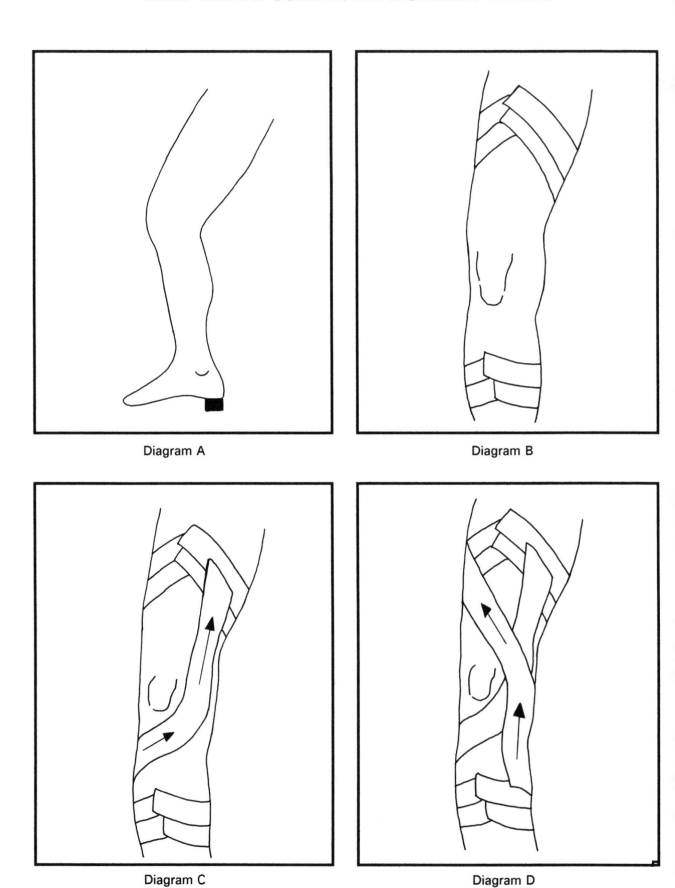

Diagram A

Diagram B

Diagram C

Diagram D

KNEE- MEDIAL COLLATERAL LIGAMENT TAPING

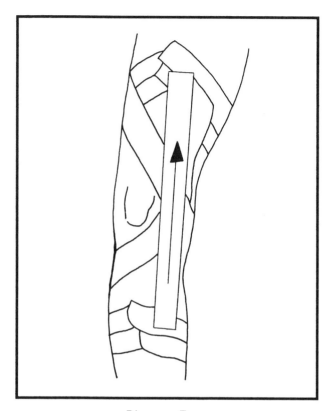

Diagram E

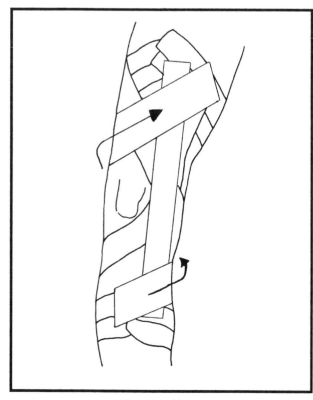

Diagram F

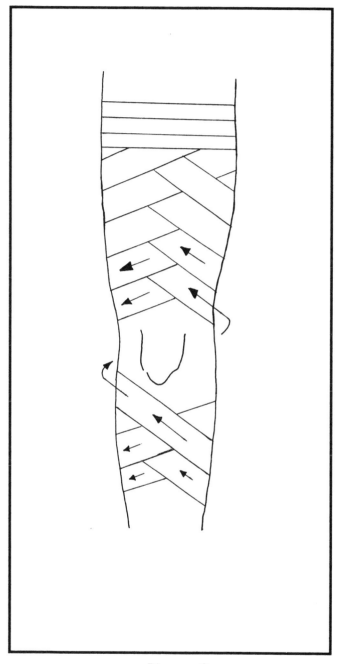

Diagram G

KNEE (HYPEREXTENSION)

PURPOSE: - To prevent hyperextension of the knee in order to provide support for a sprained posterior capsule, a lax anterior cruciate ligament or strained lower hamstring tendons.

SUPPLIES: - 3" elastic tape
- 1 1/2" white adhesive tape
- gauze pads
- skin lubricant
- pro- wrap
- tuff- skin spray
- heel & lace pads
- 6" tensor bandages (2)

IMPORTANT TEACHING POINTS:

**SKIN PREPARATION
        AND
BODY POSITIONING**

- Shave the thigh and lower leg.

- Spray the entire knee with tuff- skin.

- Apply a lubricated heel & lace pad to the back of the knee to prevent irritation.

- Secure the heel & lace pad with pro- wrap starting just above the calf and finishing mid thigh.

- Position the limb by placing a roll of 1 1/2" white adhesive tape under the athlete's heel.

- Have the athlete internally rotate his or her lower leg so that the toes face inwards.

ANCHORS

- Apply two, 3" elastic tape anchors to the upper thigh and overlap each one by half the width of the tape. By sure to have the athlete contract the thigh muscles (See Diagram B).

- Apply two, 3 " elastic tape anchors around the lower leg.

- Position the first strip below the belly of the calf and the second one mid belly.

- These strips should overlap each other by half the width of the tape.

- Have the athlete contract the calf muscles before securing these strips.

CHECKREIN FORMATION

- Measure the distance from one anchor to another by using the white adhesive tape. Lay this strip on a table and add four more to it to create a fan shaped checkrein. Secure a 1 1/ 2" white adhesive tape piece around the centre of the checkrein (See Diagram D).

CLOSURES

- Position the pre- formed checkrein on the back of the leg (See Diagram D). Secure the lower leg first with two, 3" elastic tape strips (See Diagram E).

- Now secure the checkrein on the thigh by using five, 3" elastic tape closures. Overlap these strips by half the width of the tape.

- Use two six inch tensor bandages to secure the 3" elastic tape closures. Make sure these tensor bandages start at the calf and work up to the top of the thigh. The tensor bandages should cover the entire leg. Secure the tensor bandage at the upper thigh with two 1 1/ 2" white adhesive tape strips.

- Check the function of the tape job. If the checkrein is too loose, fold the centre of the fan onto itself and then re- secure it with two strips of 1 1/ 2" white adhesive tape.

OPTION CLOSURE - To add more support to the knee- hyperextension technique, add the derotation strip as found in the knee- medial collateral ligament taping procedure (See derotation strips section). This derotation strip is applied immediately after the anchors. Then complete the knee- hyperextension technique as shown.

KNEE (HYPEREXTENSION)

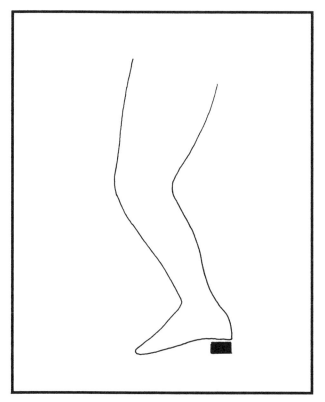

Diagram A

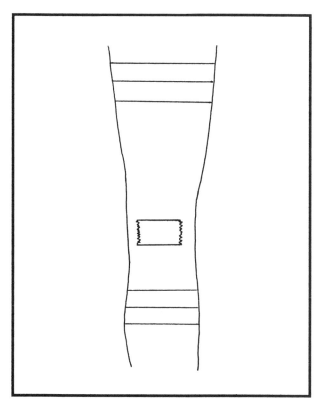

Diagram B

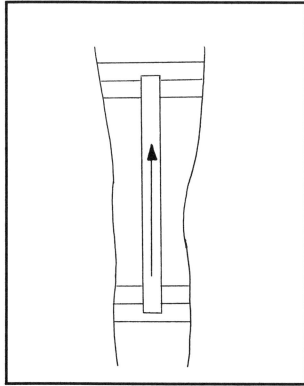

Diagram C

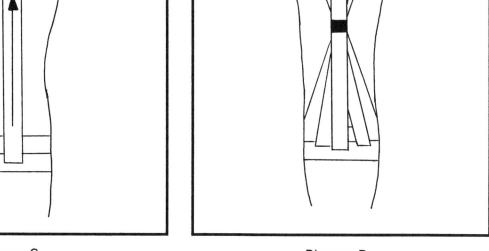

Diagram D

KNEE (HYPEREXTENSION)

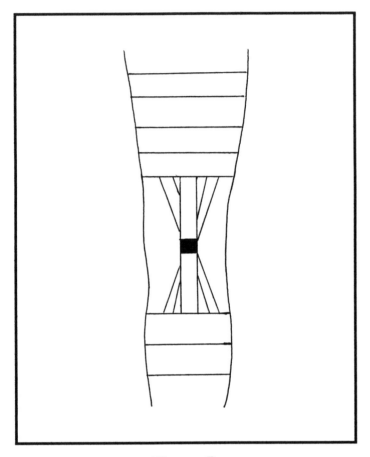

Diagram E

PATELLA TENDON TAPING

PURPOSE: - To provide support to the patella tendon and to take stress off the patella tendon insertion.

SUPPLIES: - 1 1/ 2" white adhesive tape
- tuff-skin spray
- one heel & lace pad
- foam (3/ 8" thick X 1/ 2" wide X 2" long)
- skin lubricant

IMPORTANT TEACHING POINTS:

SKIN PREPARATION

- Shave a small strip on the front and back of the knee on a horizontal line around the area of discomfort.

- Spray the front and back of the knee with tuff- skin.

- Cut the lubricated heel & lace pad in half and place the two sections behind the knee.

BODY POSITIONING

- Position the athlete with the leg slightly bent supporting the heel with a 1 1/ 2" roll of white adhesive tape (See Diagram A).

SUPPORT TECHNIQUE

- Place the foam over the area of the tendon that requires support.

- Secure a 1 1/ 2" white adhesive tape strip that goes around the patella tendon and the back of the knee.

- Repeat the horizontal closure piece again, then secure the strip on the front of the knee.

- Be sure the athlete can do a full squat and that the tape is not too tight.

61

PATELLA TENDON TAPING

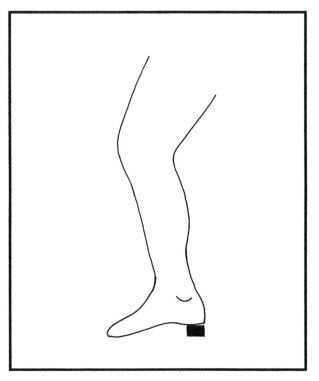

Diagram A

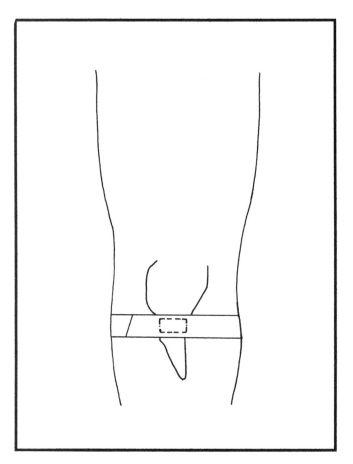

Diagram B

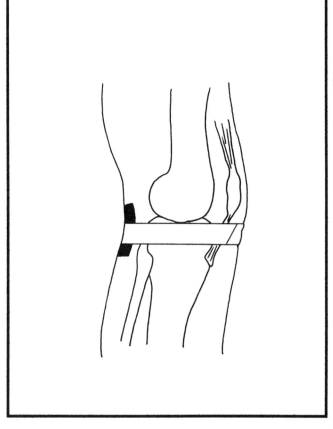

Diagram C

PATELLA- STABILIZING SUPPORT

PURPOSE: - To prevent the patella from tracking laterally, or from subluxing or dislocating.

SUPPLIES: - 3" non tearing elastic tape
- tuff- skin spray
- heel & lace pads
- 1 1/ 2" elastic tape
- 1 1/ 2" white adhesive tape
- skin lubricant

IMPORTANT TEACHING POINTS:

**SKIN PREPARATION
       AND
BODY POSITIONING**

- Shave the hair from just above and below the knee cap.

- Spray the front and back of the knee with tuff- skin.

- Position the athlete by placing a 1 1/ 2" roll of white adhesive tape under the heel (See Diagram A).

- Place two lubricated heel and lace pads on the back of the knee for protection.

SUPPORT TECHNIQUE

- Create a patella stabilizing strip from 3" elastic tape by cutting one end of the tape into two equal sections. The cut should be about 6 " deep (See Diagram B).

- Place the 6 " spilt ends on the inside of the knee so that they surround the inside of the knee cap (See Diagram C).

- Roll the tape around the back of the knee, over the heel & lace pads and up to the lateral side of the knee cap.

- Advance the elastic tape 6" beyond the outside edge of the knee cap, then cut the tape.

- Divide the end into two equal sections then
  cut it back to the outside edge of the
  knee cap.

- Move the lower strip upwards to be applied
  to the top of the knee cap. Move the
  upper strip downwards and secure below the
  knee cap (See Diagram D).

- This final step prevents possible ripping
  along the seams.

CLOSURES

- Apply a continuous strip of 1 1/ 2" elastic tape
  that will cover the skin above the knee cap.
  This same strip must continue from the
  inside and outside of the thigh to cross
  down behind the knee (See Diagram E).
  This continuous strip will eventually
  overlap on the patella tendon.

- Add a 1 1/ 2" white adhesive tape strip
  horizontally below the knee cap to secure
  the continuous elastic tape " X " strip
  (See Diagram F).

PATELLA : STABILIZING SUPPORT

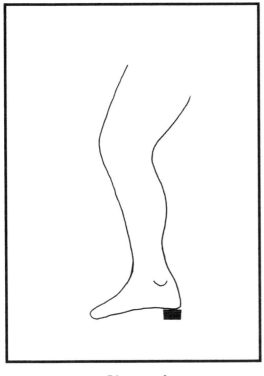

Diagram A

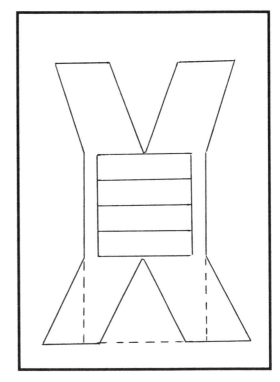

Diagram B

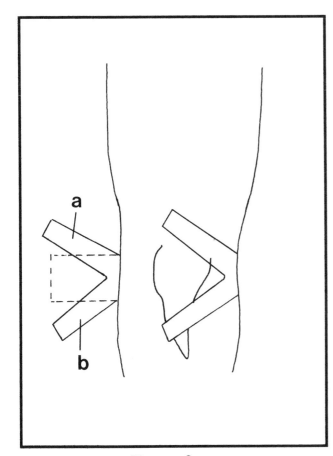

Diagram C

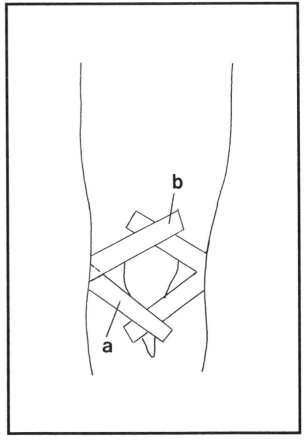

Diagram D

PATELLA : STABILIZING SUPPORT

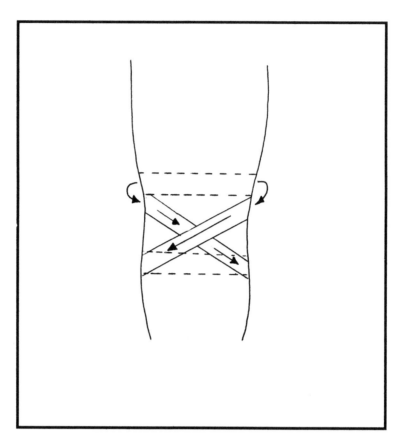

Diagram E

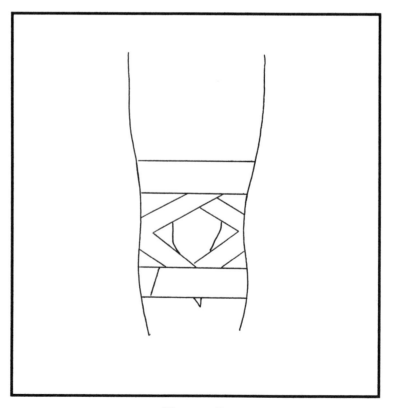

Diagram F

Chapter 4

QUADRICEPS- SUPPORT FOR A STRAIN/ CONTUSION

PURPOSE: - To provide compression to a strain or a contusion to the quadriceps muscles in the acute stage.

SUPPLIES: - 1 1/2" white adhesive tape
- tuff-skin spray
- 6" tensor bandage
- 2" white adhesive tape
- protective foam pad (medium density)

IMPORTANT TEACHING POINTS:

**SKIN PREPARATION
AND
BODY POSITIONING**

- Position the athlete by placing a 1 1/2" roll of white adhesive tape under the heel (See Diagram A).

- Shave the hair from the front of the thigh.

- Spray the thigh with tuff- skin.

ANCHORS

- Secure one 2" white adhesive tape strip on the outside of the thigh and one on the inside of the thigh (See Diagram B).

SUPPORT TECHNIQUE

- Start the 1 1/2" white adhesive tape strips below the area of injury on the inner thigh, moving upwards on a 45 degree angle (See Diagram C).

- The next support strip starts on the outside anchor of the front of the thigh. From here the strip travels upwards on a 45 degree angle.

- Repeat the strips while overlapping by half the width of the tape until the area is fully covered (See Diagram D).

- These support strips do not go entirely
  around the thigh (See Diagram E).

CLOSURES

- Close the entire tape job with a 6" tensor bandage.

- Start applying the tensor below the injury
  and then work upwards with a " TUG " on
  a 45 degree angle. Now spiral around
  the thigh and work the tensor downwards
  with a " TUG " on a 45 degree angle
  (See Diagram F).

- Repeat the above procedure to create a
  herring bone pattern (See Diagram F).

- Secure the wrap with three clips. Do not
  finish the clips on the inside of the leg
  as they could rub and cut the opposite leg
  or just pop off. Secure the wrap with two
  or three 2" white adhesive tape strips
  overlapping by half the tape width (See
  Diagram F).

QUADRICEPS- SUPPORT DUE TO A STRAIN/ CONTUSION

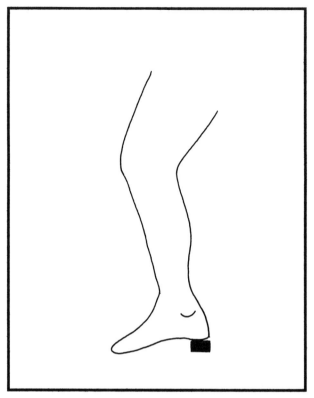

Diagram A

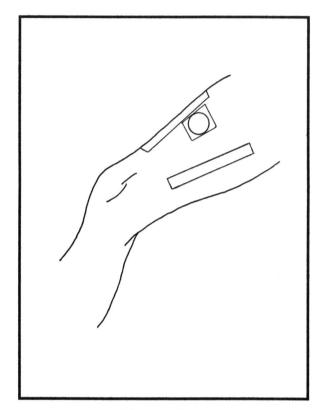

Diagram B

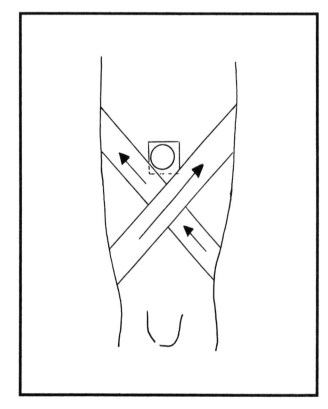

Diagram C

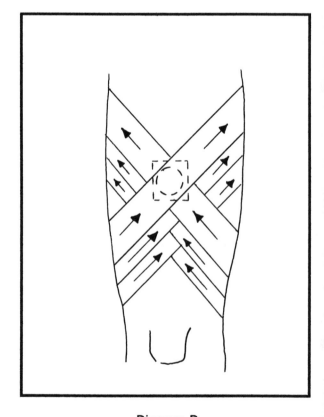

Diagram D

QUADRICEPS- SUPPORT DUE TO A STRAIN/ CONTUSION

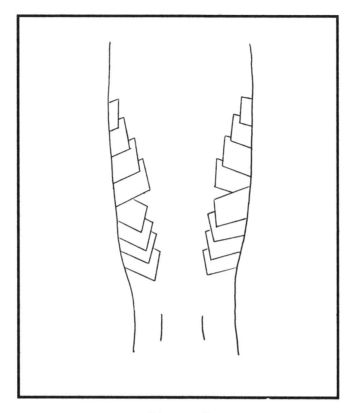

Diagram E

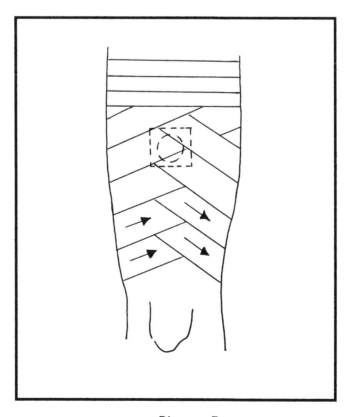

Diagram F

QUADRICEPS- SUPPORT FOR A STRAIN/ CONTUSION
(OPTION)

PURPOSE: - To provide support to the quadriceps muscles. This technique may be used as an option.

SUPPLIES: - tuff- skin spray
- 1 1/2" white adhesive tape
- pro- wrap
- 3" elastic tape (as an option for a tensor bandage)
- 6" tensor wrap
- 2" white adhesive tape
- protective foam pad (medium density)

IMPORTANT TEACHING POINTS:

SKIN PREPARATION
AND
BODY POSITIONING

- Shave the front of the thigh.

- Apply the tuff- skin to the front and back of the thigh.

- The athlete should be positioned so that the knee is bent to approximately a 30 degree angle. Position the athlete by placing a 1 1/ 2" roll of white adhesive tape under the heel (See Diagram A).

SUPPORT TECHNIQUE

- Apply four 1 1/ 2" white adhesive tape strips (rolled sticky side out) over the area to be protected (See Diagram B). These strips will help hold the pad and tensor from sliding down the leg during activity.

- Apply a pad over the area to be protected (3/ 8" thick, medium density foam as a minimum requirement- See Diagram C).

CLOSURES

- Close the entire tape job with a 6"
  tensor.

- Start applying the tensor below the area
  to be supported, then work upwards with a
  " TUG " on a 45 degree angle. Now spiral
  around the thigh and work the tensor
  downwards with a " TUG " on a
  45 degree angle. Repeat this up and down
  configuration to create a herring bone
  pattern (See Diagram D). Secure the wrap
  on the upper thigh with two clips (Do not
  finish the clips on the inside of the thigh
  as they could cut the opposite thigh or
  just pop off).

- Secure the wrap with two 2" strips of
  white adhesive tape while the athlete contracts
  the thigh muscles (See Diagram D).

QUADRICEPS- SUPPORT DUE TO STRAIN/ CONTUSION
(OPTION)

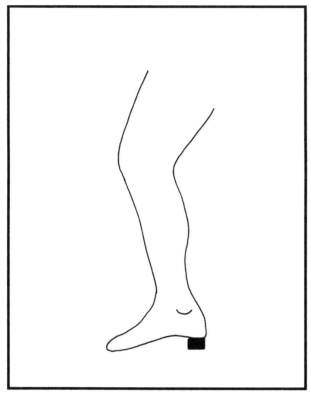

Diagram A

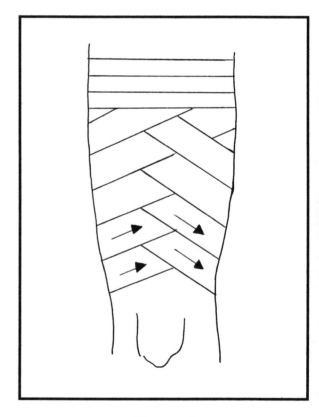

Diagram B

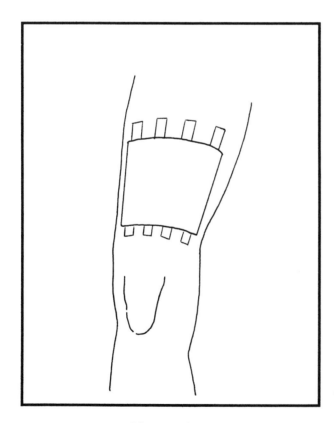

Diagram C

Diagram D

HAMSTRING- SUPPORT FOR A STRAIN/ CONTUSION

PURPOSE: - To provide compression to a strain or a contusion in the acute stage.

SUPPLIES: - tuff- skin spray
- pressure pad
- 1 1/ 2" white adhesive tape
- 6" tensor bandage
- 2" white adhesive tape

IMPORTANT TEACHING POINTS:

SKIN PREPARATION **AND** **BODY POSITIONING**	- Have the athlete lie on their stomach.
	- Shave hair from the back of the thigh.
	- Spray the thigh with tuff- skin.
	- Apply a pressure pad over the area of injury.

ANCHORS	- Secure one 2" white adhesive strip on the outside and one 2" strip on the inside of the back of the thigh (See Diagram A).

SUPPORT TECHNIQUE	- Begin the first compression strip starting below the area of injury on the inner back of the thigh going upwards on a 45 degree angle (See Diagram B).
	- The next support strip starts on the outside anchor of the back of the thigh. From here the strip travels upwards to the inside of the thigh on a 45 degree angle.
	- Repeat the above strips while overlapping by half the width of the tape until the area is fully covered (See Diagram C).
	- The tape strips do not go completely around the thigh (See Diagram D).

CLOSURES

- Close the entire tape job with a 6" tensor.

- Start applying the tensor below the injury and then work upwards with a " TUG " on a 45 degree angle. Now spiral around the thigh and work the tensor downwards with a " TUG " on a 45 degree angle as well.

- Repeat this up and down configuration to create a herring bone pattern (See Diagram E).

- Secure the wrap with three clips. (Do not finish the clips on the inside of the leg as they could rub and cut the opposite leg or just pop off). Secure the wrap with two or three 2" strips of white adhesive tape (See Diagram E).

HAMSTRING- SUPPORT DUE TO STRAIN/ CONTUSION

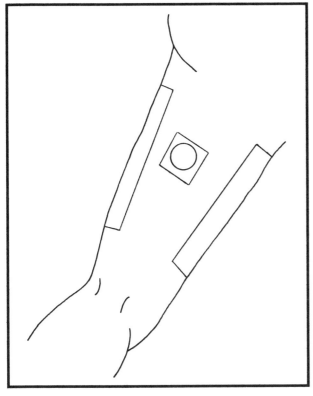

Diagram A

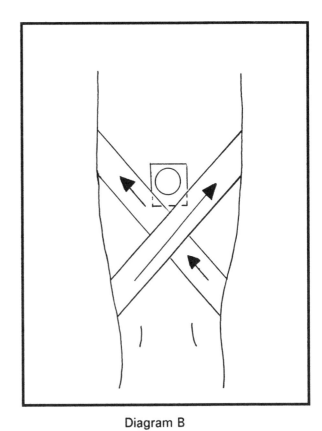

Diagram B

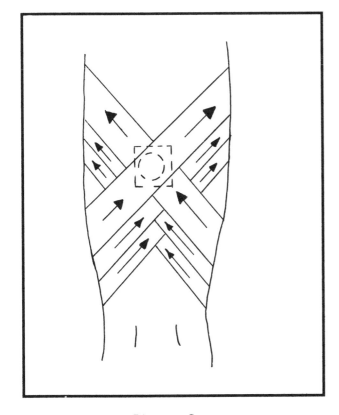

Diagram C

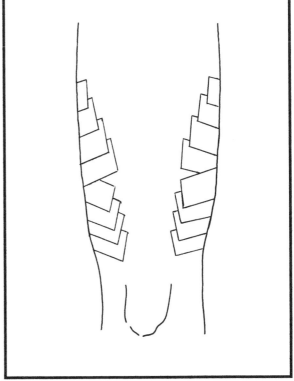

Diagram D

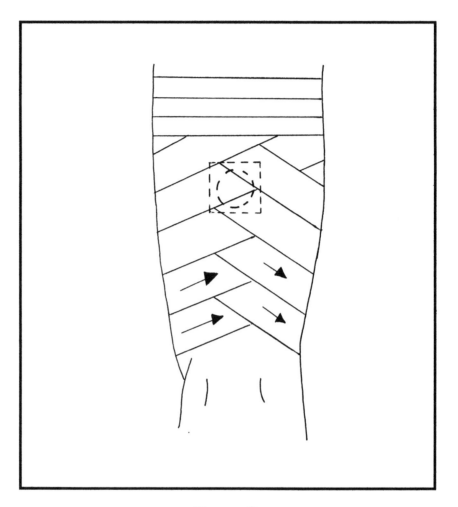

Diagram E

GROIN WRAP

PURPOSE: - To provide support for a hip flexor and/ or adductor strain.

SUPPLIES: - 6" double length tensor
- 2" white adhesive tape
- tuff- skin spray

IMPORTANT TEACHING POINTS:

**SKIN PREPARATION
AND
BODY POSITIONING**

- Spray the thigh with tuff-skin.

- Position the athlete by placing a 1 1/ 2" roll of adhesive tape under the heel. The knee should be bent slightly (See Diagram A).

- Rotate the lower leg inwards slighly.

SUPPORT TECHNIQUE

- Secure the wrap mid- thigh while wrapping towards the inner thigh. Spiral around the thigh twice then proceed upwards with a quick tug on the wrap (See Diagram B and Diagram C).

- Carry the wrap around the back, level with the top of the hip bone (See Diagram C).

- Travel downwards (See Diagram D) and around the thigh.

CLOSURES

- Repeat this figure 8 procedure then secure the wrap on the upper thigh with 2" white adhesive tape over the tensor clips (See Diagram E).

- When finished, the support technique should help spring the thigh upwards. It will also limit how far the athlete can abduct and externally rotate his/ her thigh.

CLOSURE OPTION

- Cover the entire procedure with one 3" elastic tape figure 8 by starting and finishing at the thigh. Secure the elastic tape with two 2" white adhesive tape strips. Be sure to have the athlete contract the thigh muscles before securing the white adhesive tape.

GROIN WRAP

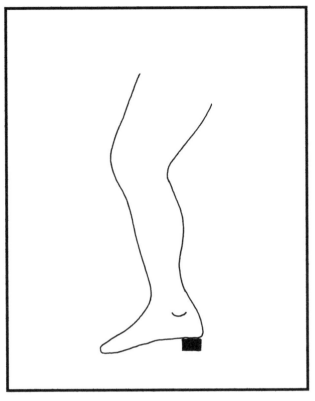

Diagram A

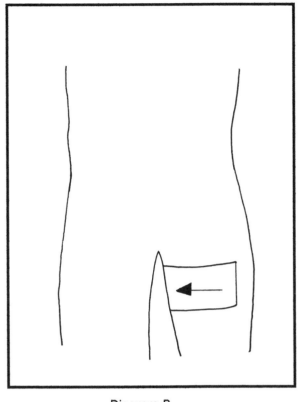

Diagram B

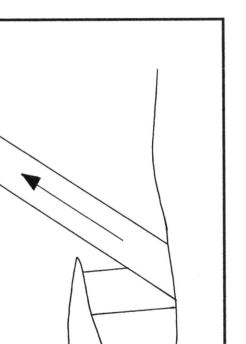

Diagram C

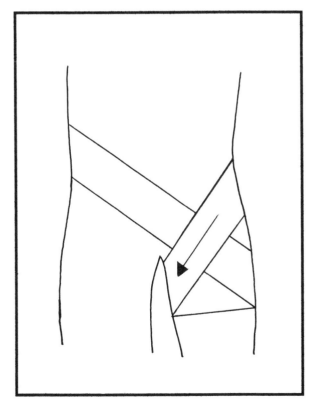

Diagram D

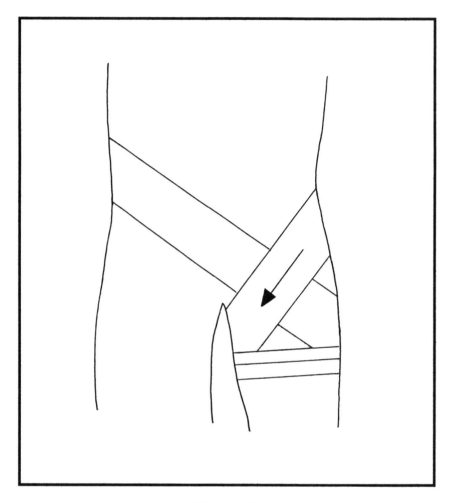

Diagram E

Chapter 5

SHOULDER: AC JOINT SUPPORT

PURPOSE: - To provide support to an acromio clavicular (AC) joint.

SUPPLIES: - tuff- skin spray
- felt or adhesive foam (1/ 2" thick)
- 3" elastic tape
- heel & lace pads
- 2" elastic tape
- 1 1/ 2" white adhesive tape
- band- aids (2 knuckle)
- skin lubricant

IMPORTANT TEACHING POINTS:

**SKIN PREPARATION
AND
BODY POSITIONING**

- Shave the area around the chest and arm prior to taping.

- Spray the arm and chest with tuff-skin.

- Cover the nipples with heel and lace pads or with a band- aid and some skin lubricant.

- The arm should be supported on a table.

- Apply a donut pad over the AC joint (See diagram A).

ANCHORS

- Apply an anchor from the nipple, passing upwards over the clavicle and then down to the shoulder blade (See Diagram A).

- Apply a 3" elastic tape anchor over the biceps muscle (mid upper arm). Have the athlete tighten the muscle before securing the tape.

- Apply a 3" elastic tape anchor around the chest. Be sure to have the athlete inhale before securing the tape (See Diagram A).

SUPPORT TECHNIQUE

- The support strips should begin on the outer part of the back of the arm then work upwards to end on the front of the chest.

- The next strip should begin on the front of the arm while crossing over the first support strip to end on the shoulder blade. This will create an " X " pattern over the AC joint.

- Repeat the above " X " pattern until the AC joint is covered (See Diagram B).

- Usually three to four strips going in each direction is adequate.

CLOSURES

- Close biceps with two 1 1/ 2" adhesive tape strips. Be sure to have the athlete flex the arm before closing the strips.

- Close the area above the nipple by using 2" elastic tape strips passing upwards from the nipple and finishing on the shoulder blade anchor. Repeat three times and overlap each strip by half the width of the tape (See Diagram C).

- Apply three 1 1/ 2" white adhesive tape strip closures which start at the nipple and go horizontally around the chest to finish at the shoulder blade. Overlap each strip by one half the width of the tape (See Diagram C).

- Finish closing by using 3" elastic tape around the chest. Have the athlete inhale before securing the tape closure (See Diagram D).

- Secure the end of the tape with three 1 1/ 2" white adhesive tape strips (See Diagram D).

- A tight fitting shirt should be worn by the athlete to keep this support technique in place.

SHOULDER: AC JOINT SUPPORT

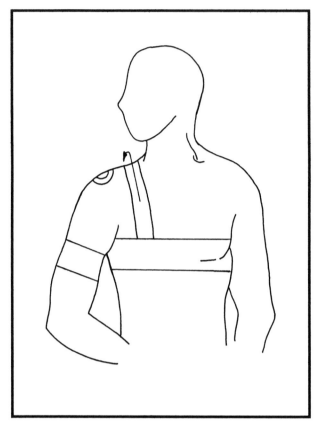

Diagram A

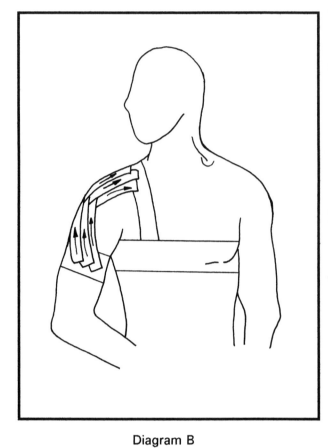

Diagram B

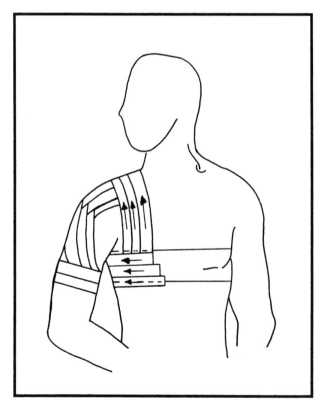

Diagram C

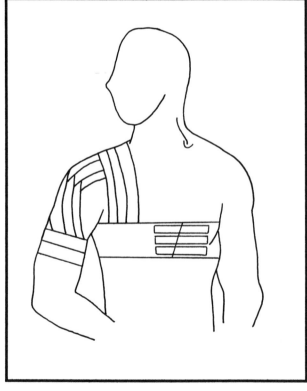

Diagram D

SHOULDER- SPICA WRAP

PURPOSE: - To prevent abduction and external rotation of the shoulder through the use of a double length tensor.

SUPPLIES: - tuff- skin spray
- 6" double length tensor wrap
- 1 1/ 2" white adhesive tape

IMPORTANT TEACHING POINTS:

SKIN PREPARATION
AND

BODY POSITIONING

- Position the athlete with their arm internally rotated (as if their hand were in their back pocket - See Diagram C).

- Cover the nipple with skin lube and a band- aid.

- Have the athlete tighten upper arm muscles during the wrap procedure.

- Spray the arm and chest lightly with tuff-skin.

ANCHOR
SUPPORT TECHNIQUE
AND
CLOSURES

- Begin the wrap by securing it around the biceps (See Diagram A). The wrap must start on the outside of the arm, wrap inwards under the arm pit then carry outwards and around the arm again. The wrap should now continue across the chest, under the opposite arm and then traverse upwards around affected shoulder again (See Diagram C).

- Repeat this procedure then clip the tensor at the arm.

- Try to finish the clips on the biceps and then cover with two 1 1/ 2" white adhesive tape strips (See Diagram E). Make sure to contract biceps muscles prior to applying the closures.

- Do not finish the tensor wrap so that the clips are next to the chest. The clips could come undone or injure the skin (See Diagram D).

SHOULDER- SPICA WRAP

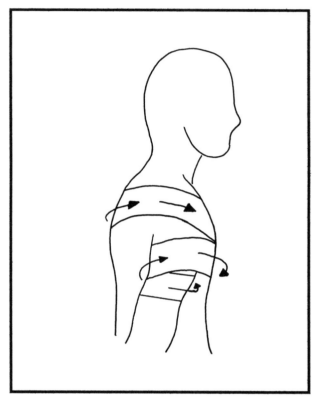

Diagram A

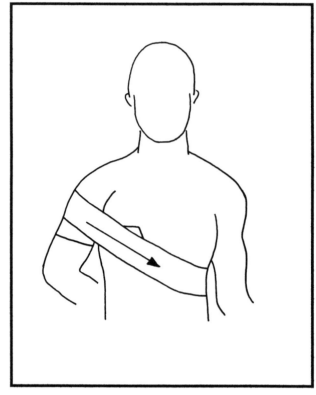

Diagram B

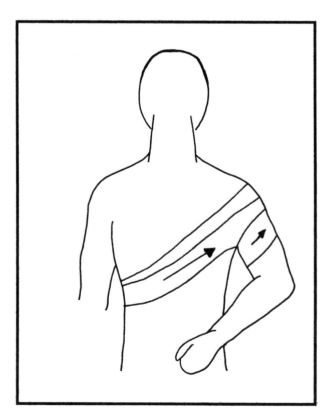

Diagram C

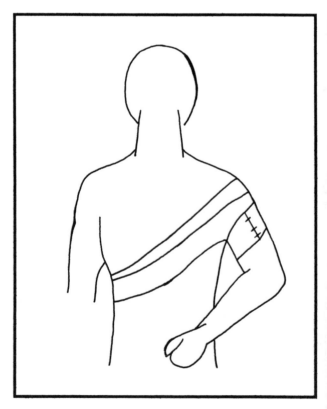

Diagram D

SHOULDER- SPICA WRAP

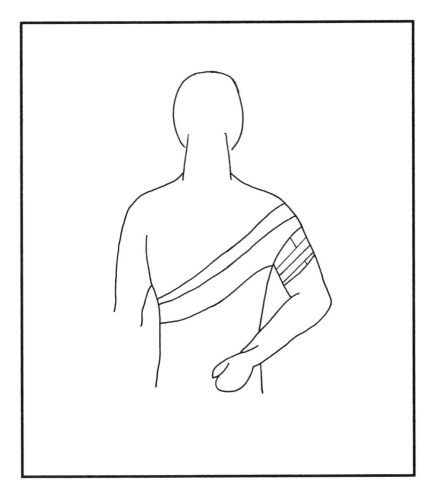

Diagram E

SHOULDER TAPING- TO PREVENT ANTERIOR DISLOCATION

PURPOSE: - To provide support for the Gleno- Humeral joint by limiting abduction and external rotation.

SUPPLIES: - tuff- skin spray
- 3" elastic tape
- 1 1/ 2" white adhesive tape

IMPORTANT TEACHING POINTS:

SKIN PREPARATION
         AND
BODY POSITIONING

- The arm and chest should first be shaved and then sprayed with tuff- skin.

- The athlete should be positioned such that his/ her arm is internally rotated, (as if their hand were in their backpocket).

ANCHORS

- Secure one 3" elastic tape anchor around the biceps while having the athlete tighten the muscle (See Diagram A).

- Secure one 3" elastic tape anchor around the chest. The athlete must inhale first before securing the tape (See Diagram A).

SUPPORT TECHNIQUE

- Begin a 3" elastic tape support strip mid- chest then travel horizontally around the chest and the affected arm to finish near the beginning of the strip (See Diagram B). Pinch the tape together between the arm and the chest.

CLOSURES

- Close the support technique by starting
  on the outside of the arm (See Diagram C). Now
  travel horizontally across the chest, behind the
  back and around the affected arm again.
  Finish this strip just near the side of the chest
  wall (See Diagram C).

- Pinch the tape together between the arm and
  chest again. Wrap several 1 1/ 2"
  white adhesive strips around the checkrein
  that has been established between the
  arm and the chest (See Diagram C).

SHOULDER TAPING- TO PREVENT ANTERIOR DISLOCATION

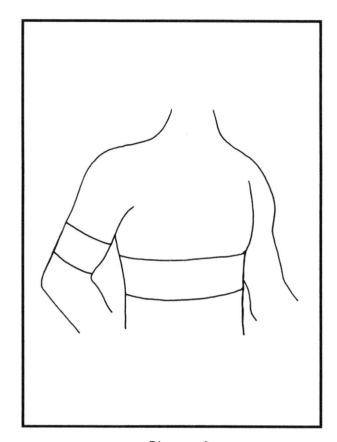

Diagram A

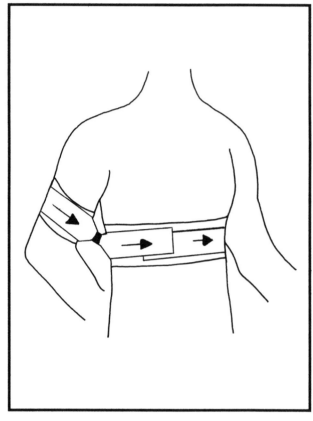

Diagram B

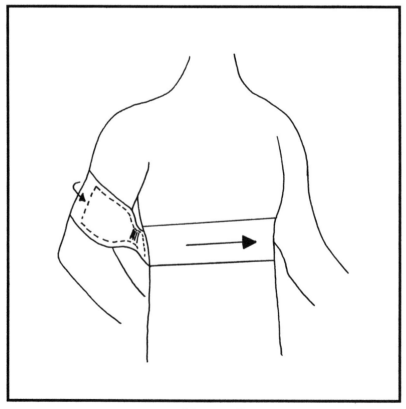

Diagram C

92

Chapter 6

ELBOW (HYPEREXTENSION)

PURPOSE: - To prevent the elbow from hyperextending.

SUPPLIES: - tuff- skin spray
- 1 1/ 2" white adhesive tape
- 3" elastic tape
- skin lubricant

IMPORTANT TEACHING POINTS:

SKIN PREPARATION **AND** **BODY POSITIONING**	- Shave the upper and lower arm. - Spray the upper and lower arm with tuff- skin. - Position the elbow in a slightly bent position.

ANCHORS	- Apply two 1 1/ 2" adhesive tape anchors around the mid forearm. Overlap each strip by half the width of the tape. Make sure the athlete opens his/ her fingers fully and tightens forearm musculature (See Diagram A). - Apply two 3" elastic tape anchors around the biceps muscle. The first anchor goes around the mid biceps and the second anchor goes above the biceps. Overlap each piece by half the width of the tape. Have the athlete contract the biceps before securing the anchors (See Diagram A).

CHECKREIN FORMATION	- Once the painfree angle of the elbow has been established, measure the distance from one anchor to another by using the white adhesive tape. Lay this strip on a table and add six more to it to create a fan shaped checkrein. Secure a 1 1/ 2" white adhesive tape piece around the centre of the checkrein (See Diagram B).

CLOSURES

- Position the pre- formed checkrein
  (See Diagram C). Secure the forearm first
  with two 1 1/ 2" white adhesive tape
  strips (See Diagram D).

- Now secure the checkrein on the biceps.
  Use one 3" elastic tape piece over the mid
  belly area. Close the area beyond the biceps
  muscle with one 2" adhesive tape strip.
  Have the athlete contract the biceps
  before applying both closures (See Diagram D).

ELBOW (HYPEREXTENSION)

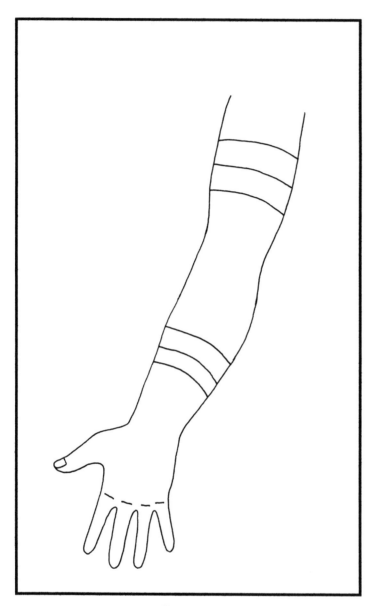

Diagram A

Diagram B

ELBOW (HYPEREXTENSION)

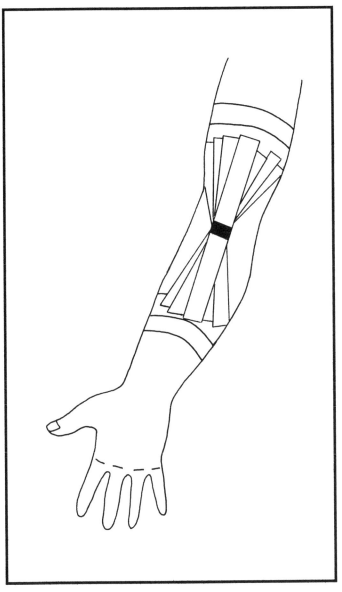

Diagram C

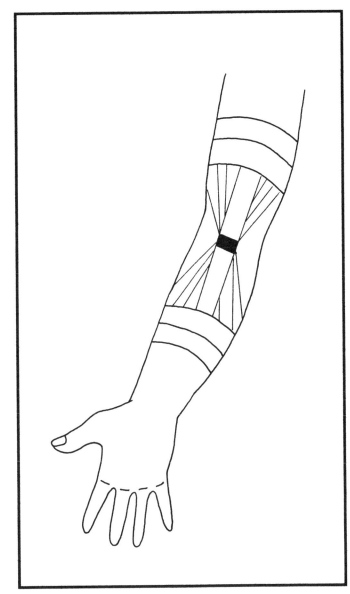

Diagram D

WRIST- HYPEREXTENSION SUPPORT

PURPOSE: - To prevent excessive wrist extension.

SUPPLIES: - tuff- skin spray
- 1 1/ 2" white adhesive tape
- 1/ 2" white adhesive tape

IMPORTANT TEACHING POINTS:

**SKIN PREPARATION
AND
BODY POSITIONING**

- Shave the arm of the forearm to be taped.

- Spray the forearm and hand with tuff- skin.

- Have the athlete hold the wrist in a straight position (neutral) with the fingers spread apart.

- Place the athlete's fingers on your stomach to prevent any movement of the wrist during the taping procedure.

ANCHORS

- Use 1 1/ 2" white adhesive tape to create three wrist anchors. The first wrist anchor starts at the crease in the wrist. The other two anchors continue up the forearm from here and are overlapped by half the width of the tape.

- The fourth hand anchor starts and finishes on the back of the hand (See Diagram A).

- Be sure to fold the white adhesive tape when going over the web of the thumb.

- Do not cover the knuckles of the fingers as the athlete should be able to make a fist.

- The fifth hand anchor starts at the wrist, on a slight angle. This piece travels down the inside of the wrist, over the back of the hand and down the palm and finishes at the base of the thumb (See Diagram B). Be sure to fold the edges of the tape over when crossing the web of the thumb.

- Apply one last anchor (sixth) at the base of the thumb, starting on the back of the hand, on the fifth anchor and finishing in the palm, on anchor # 5 (See Diagram C).

CHECKREIN SUPPORT

- Measure the required length of the checkrein by measuring from one anchor to the other.

- Once the length has been established, form an " X " on top of the piece of 1 1/2" white adhesive tape (See Diagram D).

CLOSURES

- Begin the close up of the tape job by repeating the fourth anchor. This will be called closure number one (C1).

- Repeat the fifth hand anchor. This will be called closure number two (C2).

- Now take the checkrein and pull the wrist into slight flexion while securing the checkrein onto the forearm (See Diagram D).

- Secure the forearm with 3 overlapping closure strips of 1 1/2" white adhesive tape (C3, C4, C5).

- Now check the function of the wrist.

OPTION

- Secure one or two 1/2" white adhesive tape strips over the crease in the wrist for extra support (See Diagram F).

WRIST- HYPEREXTENSION SUPPORT

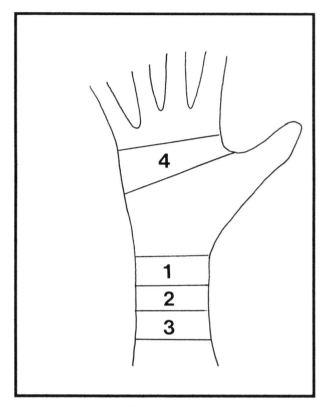

Diagram A

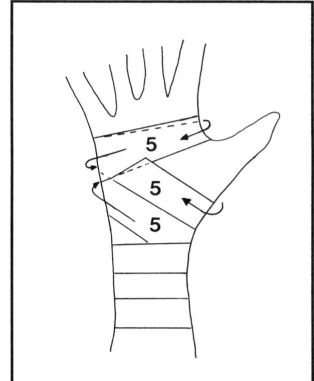

Diagram B

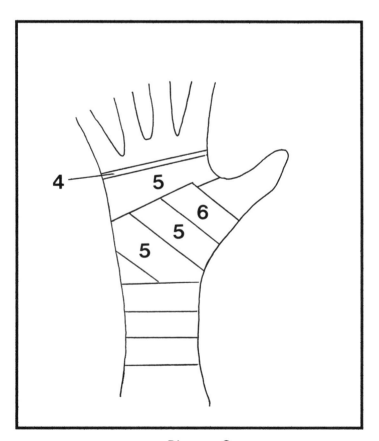

Diagram C

WRIST- HYPEREXTENSION SUPPORT

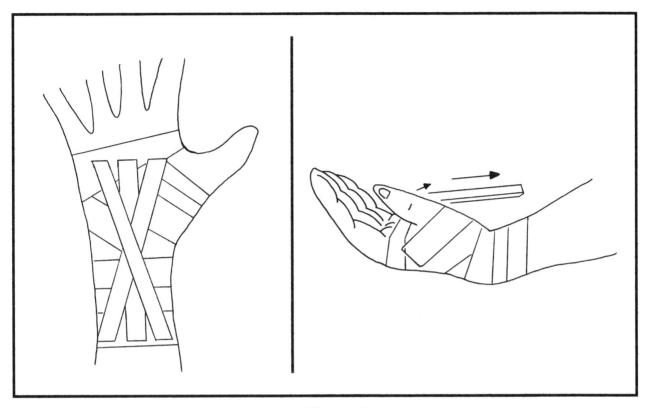

Diagram D

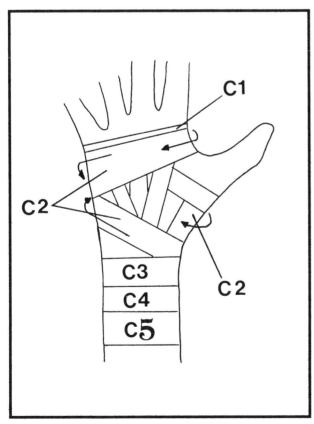

Diagram E

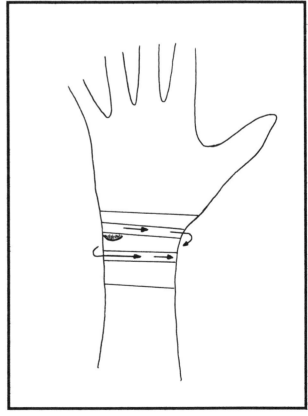

Diagram F

THUMB - HYPEREXTENSION SUPPORT

PURPOSE: - To prevent hyperextension of the thumb.

SUPPLIES: - tuff- skin spray
- 1 1/ 2" white adhesive tape

IMPORTANT TEACHING POINTS:

SKIN PREPARATION **AND** **BODY POSITIONING**	- The hand is supported on the therapist's chest
	- The thumb should be positioned in a functional position (See Diagram A).
	- Spray the entire hand with tuff- skin.

ANCHORS	- The first anchor should start on the front of the wrist (See Diagram B), wrap around the back of the hand and through the web of the thumb (See Diagram C). As the tape passes over the webbing of the thumb , you should pinch the edges to prevent the tape from cutting the skin.
	- Continue the anchor down the palm and around the wrist to finish on the front of the wrist (See Diagram C).
	- This strip can be repeated for more stability and support (optional).

HOOD FORMATION **&** **SUPPORT TECHNIQUE**	- Start the hoods on the back of the anchor at the base of the thumb, wrap around and attach onto the front of the anchor (See Diagram D).
	- Repeat these strips by continuing up the thumb and overlapping by half the width of the tape each time (See Diagram E).

- The number of hoods required will
  depend on the length of the thumb.

- Pinch the edges of the last hood piece together
  in order to help prevent hyperextension. The
  last hood piece should not interfere with bending of
  the tip of the thumb.

- The degree of hyperextension restriction
  will depend upon the positioning of the thumb.

CLOSURES

- To close, reapply the original hand anchor to
  secure the hood pieces (See Diagram F).

OPTION (HYPERABDUCTION SUPPORT)

FIGURE 8

- To prevent the thumb from opening up
  into abduction, apply two figure 8 strips
  going in the same direction (See Diagram G).
  The two strips should be continuous and should
  form a tight loop around the base of the thumb.

- Do not apply the tape too tight as it is easy to
  cut off circulation.

THUMB- HYPEREXTENSION SUPPORT

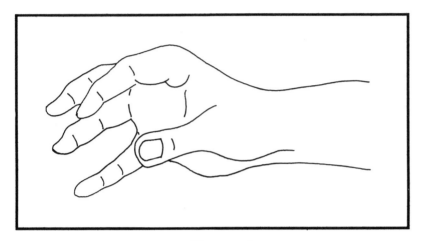

Diagram A

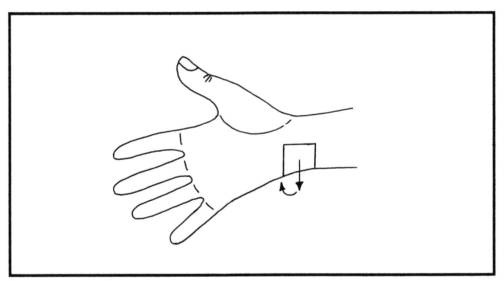

Diagram B

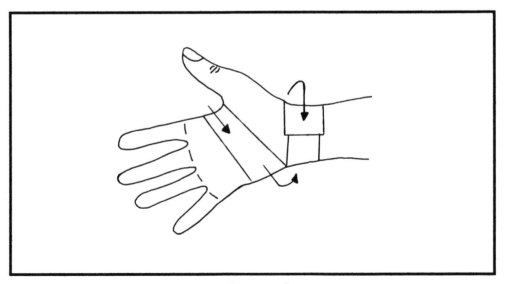

Diagram C

THUMB- HYPEREXTENSION SUPPORT

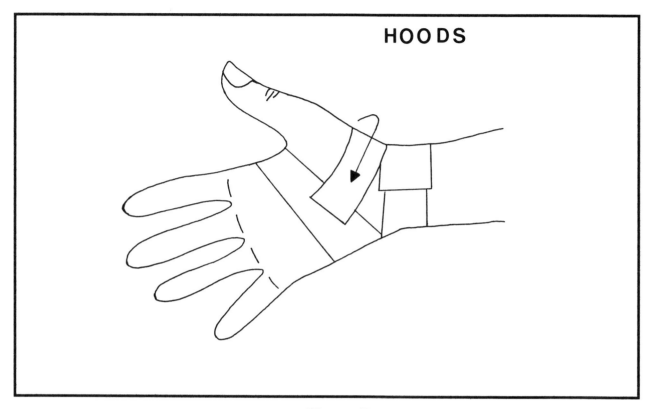

HOODS

Diagram D

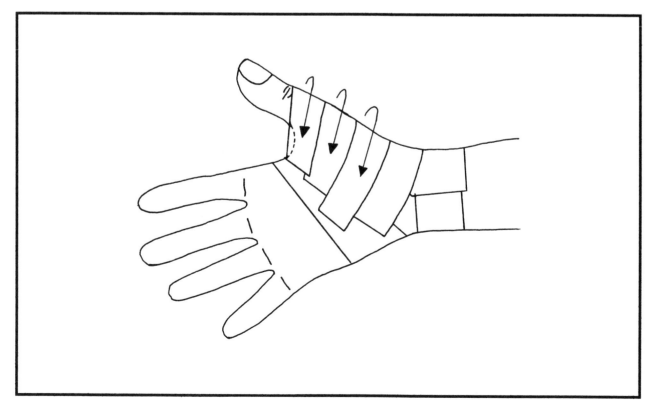

Diagram E

THUMB- HYPEREXTENSION SUPPORT

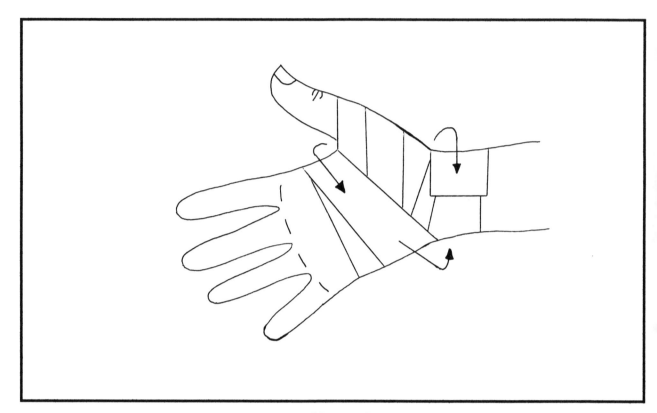

Diagram F

(OPTION- HYPERABDUCTION SUPPORT STRIPS)

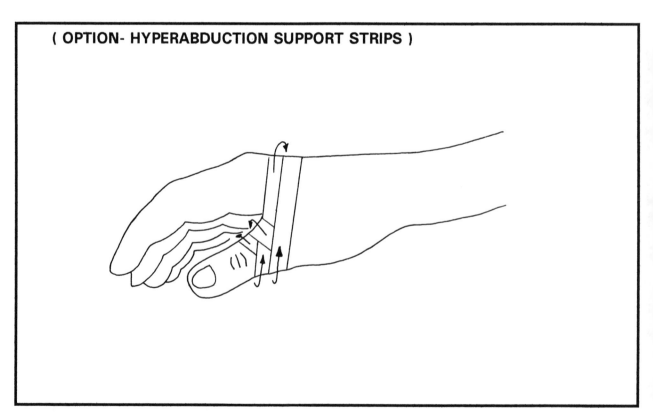

Diagram G

106

THUMB- HYPEREXTENSION (CHECKREIN METHOD)

PURPOSE: - To prevent hyperextension of the thumb.

SUPPLIES: - tuff-skin spray
   - 1" white adhesive tape

IMPORTANT TEACHING POINTS:

SKIN PREPARATION **AND** **BODY POSITIONING**	- Position the thumb in a functional painfree range of extension (See Diagram A). - Spray the thumb and index finger with tuff-skin.

ANCHORS	- Apply a 1" anchor to first digit of thumb and first digit of index finger (See Diagram A).

SUPPORT TECHNIQUE	- Secure the two digits together with a 1" white adhesive tape loop, joining the two fingers together. Pinch the tape together between the fingers to create a checkrein (See Diagram B). - Apply a final 1" tape closure over the tape that has been pinched together (See Diagram B). - Be sure that the index finger and the thumb joints can flex properly. - Check the function of the support technique.

THUMB- HYPER EXTENSION (CHECKREIN METHOD)

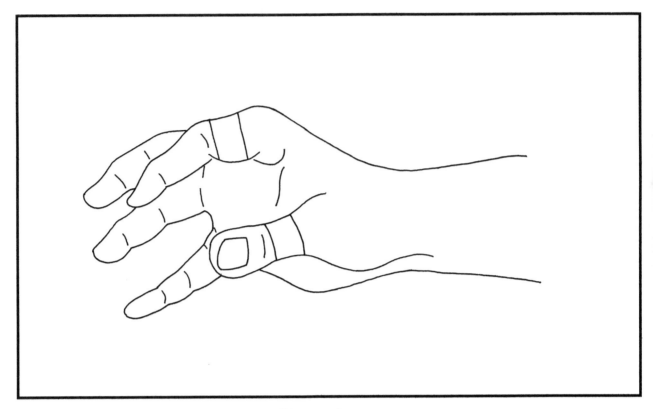

Diagram A

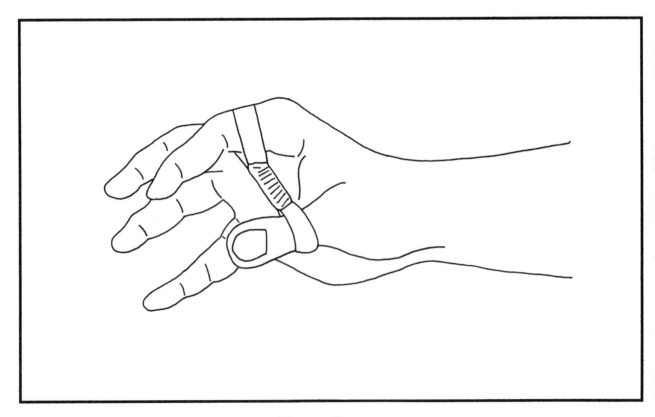

Diagram B

FINGER TAPING (BUDDY TAPING)

PURPOSE: - To immobilize an injured finger joint or
as a measure to prevent finger injury.

SUPPLIES: - tuff- skin spray
- 3" x 3" gauze pads
- 1 1/ 2" and 1" white adhesive tape

IMPORTANT TEACHING POINTS:

SKIN PREPARATION - Spray the two fingers with tuff- skin.

SUPPORT TECHNIQUE - Cut gauze, felt or foam to fit between the
injured and non injured " support " finger.

- Preference for buddy taping involves pairing
fingers # 2, # 3 and # 4, # 5 by taping above
and below the injured joint (See Diagram A).

- Finish by tearing the tape on the back of the
hand to prevent the tape from unwinding
(See Diagram A).

FINGER TAPING (BUDDY TAPING)

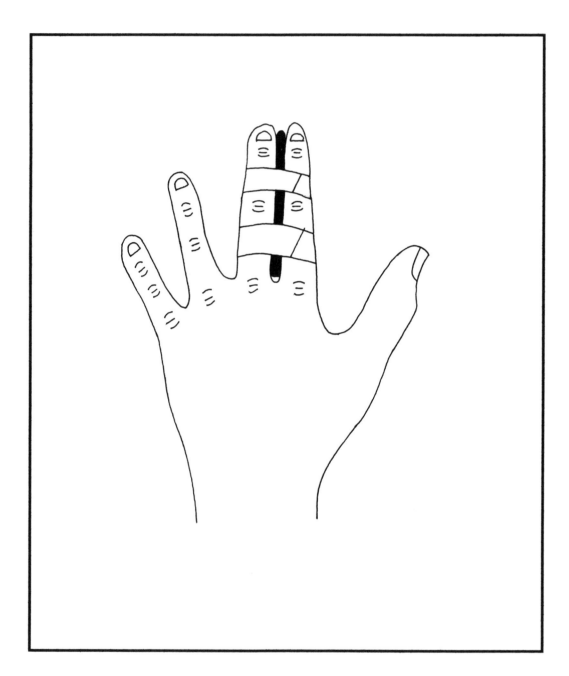

Diagram A

Chapter 7

1- APPENDIX

APPENDIX

Abduction: - The lateral movement of a limb away from the median plane of the body.

Acute: - Immediate injury onset associated with inflammation.

Adduction: - The movement of a body segment toward the median anatomical line of a nearby segment.

Anterior: - The front of the body or a body part.

Articulation: - A joint between bones.

Avulsion: - A Forcible tearing away of a part or structure i.e. A ligament from a bone.

Axilla: - Arm pit.

Bursa: - A fluid- filled sac or saclike cavity that allows a muscle or tendon to slide over bone thereby reducing friction.

Check rein: - Several strips of tape that run between upper and lower anchors. It is often shaped like an hour glass.

Chronic Injury :   - An injury showing little change or slow improvement. The opposite of acute.

Dislocation: - The displacement of one or more bones, a joint, or any organ from it's original position.

Distal: - Farthest from a center, from the midline, or from the trunk. Farthest from a point of reference (opposite of proximal).

Dorsal: - Upper surface (i.e. top of hand/ foot)

Dorsiflexion: - Moving the toe or foot, finger or wrist, toward the dorsal aspect of a nearby body segment.

Dorsum: - The back of a body part.

Edema: - Swelling as a result of the collection of fluid in the connective tissue.

Effusion: - Escape of the fluid into a cavity (such as within a joint capsule).

Epiphysis: - A growth plate.

Eversion: - Moving the soles of the feet so that they are facing away from each other.

Extension;	- Moving a body segment toward a straight line position.
Fascia:	- Fibrous membrane that covers, supports, and separates muscles.
Fascitis:	- Inflammation of fascia.
Flexion:	- Moving a body segment away from a straight line position.
Forefoot:	- The area of the foot before the toes (arch area).
Heel & Lace Pads :	- A 3" X 3" closed cell foam pad, 2 - 3 mm thick, designed to protect the skin (made by Cramer Products Inc).
Hematoma:	- A bruise - consisting of a collection of blood which is usually clotted
Hemorrhage:	- Escaping of blood through ruptured walls of blood vessels.
Hyper:	- Prefix meaning too much (i.e. hyperextension).
Hyper-Extension:	- Beyond the normal extension.
Hyperflexion:	- In excess of normal flexion.
Hypo:	- Prefix signifying a lack of or deficiency; also a position below, under or beneath.
Inferior:	- Towards the bottom of the body or body part.
Insertion:	- Muscle attachment to a bone that moves.
Inversion:	- Moving the feet so that the soles face each other.
itis :	- A suffix, an inflammation of something i.e. tendonitis
Joint Capsule:	- (articular capsule or synovial capsule)- A saclike, fibrous membrane that surrounds a joint, often including or interwoven with ligaments.
Joint Subluxation:	- Partial displacement of the articular surfaces between two or more bones.
Lateral:	- Away from the midline of the body. Pertains to the side (in relationship of position from the midline of the body).
Ligament:	- A band of flexible, tough, dense white fibrous connective tissue connecting the articular ends of the bones and sometimes enveloping them in a capsule.

113

Malleolus: - A rounded bony protuberance on each side of the ankle joint.

Medial: - Towards the midline of the body.

**Medium
Density Foam** - Similar to that found in hockey helmets

Muscle: - A tissue composed of contractile fibers or cells. A contractile organ composed of muscle tissue.

**Myositis
Ossificans:** - Inflammation of muscle, with the formation of bone tissue in it.

Neutral: - Indifferent, or neither extreme.

**Non Tearing
Tape :** - Tape that must be cut with scissors - will not tear.

Origin: - The fixed end or attachment of a muscle, ligament etc...

Palmar: - Pertaining to the palm of the hand.

Phalanges: - Bones of the fingers and toes.

Plantar: - Ventral aspect of the foot (sole of the foot).

**Plantar
Flexion:** - Moving the toe or foot toward the plantar aspect of a nearby body part. i.e. Pointing the toe and foot.

**Popliteal
Space:** - The area behind the knee joint.

Posterior: - The back of the body or a body part.

Prone: - Face- down, horizontal position of the body.

Prophylactic: - Any agent or regimen that contributes to the prevention of an injury or disease.

Pro- wrap: - A thin tearable wrap used as a protective barrier against the skin. It comes by the roll and is also know as under wrap or pre- wrap.

Proximal: - An area closest to the point of attachment, origin, or point of reference.

Separation: - Injury to a general non- movable joint (i.e. an AC Joint separation).

Spica: - Continuous strips of tape or a tensor that wrap around a joint forming a figure 8.

Sprain: - An overstress of a joint, producing a stretching or tearing of the ligaments and capsule.

Strain: - Excessive stretching or overuse of a part, as tendon or a muscle.

Superior: - Towards the top of the body or body part.

Splay: - To spread apart or move outwards.

Supine: - Lying on the back. face upwards, opposed to prone.

Tendon: - A band of dense fibrous tissue forming the termination of a muscle and attaching the latter to a bone.

Tuff-skin: - A sticky skin adherent spray made by Cramer Products Inc.

Turf- Toe :   - A toe injury resulting from the big toe being forced against the tip of the shoe. This results in excessive flexion of the big toe.

Valgus: - Position of a body part that is bent outwards away from the midline of the body.

Varus: - Position of a body part that is bent inwards toward the midline of the body.

Ventral: - Bottom surface (opposite of dorsal); near, on, or towards the belly; in man, anterior.

NOTES

NOTES

NOTES

NOTES

NOTES